TRAYS, TROLLEYS AND

THE AUTHOR

Helen M. Dickie
R.G.N., R.F.N., S.C.M.
Nurse Tutor,
Renfrew, Dumbarton and Argyll
College of Nursing and Midwifery,
Paisley.

Previously published as
Pocket Book on Tray and Trolley Setting

TRAYS, TROLLEYS AND TREATMENTS

A NURSE'S GUIDE

Helen M. Dickie

SIXTH EDITION

CHURCHILL LIVINGSTONE
EDINBURGH LONDON AND NEW YORK 1977

CHURCHILL LIVINGSTONE
Medical Division of Longman Group Limited

Distributed in the United States of America by Churchill
Livingstone Inc., 19 West 44th Street, New York, N.Y.
10036 and by associated companies, branches and
representatives throughout the world.

First Edition	1959
Second Edition	1961
Third Edition	1963
Fourth Edition	1966
Reprinted	1968
Fifth Edition	1970
Reprinted	1972
Reprinted	1974
Sixth Edition	1977
Reprinted	1979

First five editions published under the title *Pocket Book on
Tray and Trolley Setting,* by Helen M. Dickie.

ISBN 0 443 01619 4

Library of Congress Cataloging in Publication Data
Dickie, Helen McEwen.
  Trays, trolleys, and treatments.

  Fifth ed. published in 1970 under title: Pocket
book on tray and trolley setting.
  1. Nursing — Equipment and supplies. 2. Hospitals —
Furniture, equipment, etc. I. Title.
RT44.D5 1977   610.73'028   77—2195

PRINTED IN SINGAPORE
BY SINGAPORE OFFSET PRINTING PTE LTD

Preface to the Sixth Edition

In this edition I have made considerable change. The many new developments in equipment and the introduction of more efficient methods of carrying out practical procedures has necessitated major alteration to content and presentation.

Not all trays and trolleys are now illustrated as many can be prepared by simply adding to a list of basic requirements or a standard 'pack'. The continuing development of pre-packed sterilised equipment and the use of the 'composite treatment tray' supplied from a Central Sterile Supply Department has altered the pattern of tray and trolley setting.

I have therefore aimed at providing some information on trays, trolleys and treatments in as concise a form as possible and have added many illustrations which I hope will prove helpful to the practical nurse.

Clinical notes have been introduced throughout and some pages have been left for personal notes.

The chapter on sterilisation has been revised to bring it up to date with present knowledge on the subject.

The introduction of the Système International d'Unités (SI units) has also accounted for change and information which affects the nurse's practical work has been included.

It is hoped that the book in its new format will continue to prove useful.

1977   H. M. DICKIE

Preface to the First Edition

There is an old Chinese proverb which states: 'A thousand hearings are not as good as one seeing.' The subject of visual aids in teaching is receiving considerable attention to-day. No one concerned with nurse training can afford to overlook the opportunities in this field.

In compiling this little book no attempt has been made to include every tray and trolley which the nurse may require to prepare in her routine ward work. However, using the General Nursing Council (Scotland) Syllabus as a guide, I have endeavoured to include illustrations for most practical procedures carried out at the bedside.

We do well to remember the words of the International Code of Nursing Ethics – 'Service to mankind is the primary function of nurses and the reason for the existence of the nursing profession.' I trust therefore that the use of the book may not only help nurses in training to overcome some difficulties, but may result in some valuable time being saved in these days when the cry echoes through so many of our hospital wards, 'No time to nurse.' The pages which have been left throughout for notes will, I hope, serve a useful purpose.

With the existent diversity of thought on nursing procedures standardisation is not easily accomplished, but that it could be is not in doubt. In view of this diversity it has been no easy task to try to reach a point midway between over-simplification and undue elaboration, but this has been aimed at in the preparation of illustrations.

No doubt all are familiar with the fact that syringes can be sterilised by autoclaving, exposure in the hot air oven, the use of infra-red radiation or, if they are of the disposable variety, discarded after use. The administration of an enema saponis, to mention only one extremely familiar procedure, can now be carried out with the minimum of effort, time and equipment. As such advances continue, the requirements for practical procedures must of necessity change, but whatever the change in pattern may be the basic nursing needs of the patient will emerge unaltered. More advanced techniques will certainly be joined by others equally complex and requiring the intelligent co-operation of the nurse at every stage.

The fact that we are on the eve of exciting developments in the sphere of nursing in this country cannot be disputed. The rumblings of the past two decades from within the profession are gaining in momentum from those arising as a result of external pressures. In the midst of this scene of change the earnest desire of all engaged in this service to humanity is that an atmosphere may be created conducive to the patient's physical, social and spiritual well-being.

Glasgow, 1959   H. M. DICKIE

Acknowledgements

My sincere thanks to Mr R. Callander and Mr I. Ramsden of the Department of Medical Illustration, The University of Glasgow, for the excellent way in which the illustrations for this new edition have been prepared.

I am grateful to the staff of Churchill Livingstone for continued help and encouragement and also for permission to use the diagrams and text on pages 116 and 117.

I must add a word of thanks to Miss Marion McKerrow who typed the manuscript and Miss Mary Dickie for her help with reading of the proofs.

I am indebted to the many nursing students and colleagues who made helpful suggestions and offered constructive criticism during preparation of the sixth edition.

H. M. D.

Trays, Trolleys and Treatments

Bathing of patients

Trolley for bathing in bed

A large basin of water at a suitable temperature (40°C)
A bath thermometer.
Soap in a soap dish.
Two washing cloths in a receptacle.
Nail scissors in a receptacle.
A tin of talcum powder.
A jar of zinc and castor oil ointment and a wooden spatula to
    facilitate removal of ointment from jar.
A nail brush in a receptacle.
A dressing comb.
A box with disposable tissues and a disposal bag.
Two bathing sheets (terry towelling, flannelette or the patient's bed
    sheets). Always laundered after each bath.
Two bath towels and a face towel.
Clean linen for the patient and the bed.
A large jug with supply of fresh, warm water (except when it is more
    convenient to refill basin at tap).
A bucket for soiled water as required.
Appropriate bag for soiled linen.
Extra protection for the bed and floor when necessary.

Clinical notes

Patient's own toilet requisites are usually kept at the bedside. Ensure
    privacy and a draught free atmosphere.
Provide opportunity for the patient to empty his bladder before com-
    mencing the bath.
Exercise the necessary care to avoid embarrassment to the patient
    while ensuring that all areas are thoroughly washed and dried.
When the patient is able and his condition permits, he may be allowed
    to assist with the washing.
Observation and accurate reporting is important and nurse should
    note any skin rash, bruising, scars, undue redness or swelling and
    the presence of pediculi.
Any complaints of pain or impaired mobility should always be
    reported.

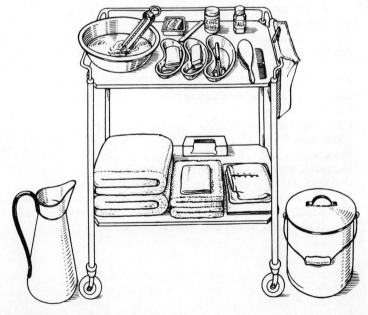

Figure 1
Trolley for bed-bathing

Care of pressure areas

Trolley for routine local treatment

A basin of warm water.

Soap in a soap dish.

Materials for cleaning areas as required, e.g. cotton wool or disposable tissues.

A disposal bag.

A disposable towel or patient's own treatment towel.

A suitable application for pressure areas, e.g. zinc and castor oil ointment, olive oil or a barrier cream.

A jug of fresh water.

A bucket for soiled water.

N.B. Local application to pressure areas must be supplementary to:

Frequent change of position, e.g. hourly or two hourly, and using a charted turning cycle when appropriate.

Attention to general cleanliness of the skin.

Ensuring a clean, dry, non-irritating bed.

Adequate nutrition of the patient.

The use of special equipment where appropriate

Alternating air pressure mattresses.

Net suspension beds.

Plastic foam mattresses.

Water beds.

Bed cradles.

Sheepskin, tubipad, foam heel rests and pads.

Overhead trapeze (especially useful in orthopaedic wards).

The skin over the following parts of the body are particularly at risk:

The occiput, scapulae, spinous processes of vertebrae and the sacrum.

The elbows, heels, ankles and femoral trochanters.

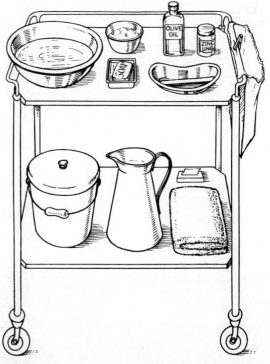

Figure 2
Trolley for local treatment of pressure areas

Example of a two hourly turning cycle

Position	Time	Nurse's signature
Left lateral	0800hrs	
	1600hrs	
	2400hrs	
Dorsal	0600hrs	
	1400hrs	
	2200hrs	
Right lateral	0400hrs	
	1200hrs	
	2000hrs	
Prone	1000hrs	
	1800hrs	
	0200hrs	

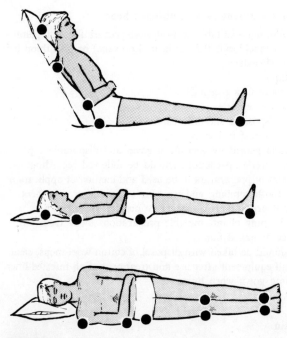

Figure 3
Areas of the body subject to special pressure

Care of the hair

1. Tray for inspection of hair and scalp

A bottle of suitable antiseptic solution, e.g. Hibitane and Cetavlon
 1:200.
A small bowl for the antiseptic solution.
A bowl with cotton wool mops.
Fine tooth comb(s) in a receptacle.
Dressing comb(s) in a receptacle.
A disposal bag for soiled cotton wool.
A plastic or disposable shoulder cape.
Polythene to protect the bed as required.
(Nurse should wear a gown for her own protection).

2. Tray for treatment of a verminous head

A bottle containing a suitable anti-infestive preparation, e.g. gamma
 benzene hexachloride 0.2 per cent (Lorexane) or malathion 0.5
 per cent (Prioderm).
A small gallipot.
A dressing comb in a receptacle.
A pipette in a receptacle.
A plastic or disposable shoulder cape.
Polythene to protect bed as required.
(Nurse protects herself by wearing a gown and disposable cap).
The manufacturer's instructions should be followed regarding:
 Amount of preparation to be used and method of application.
 Fine tooth combing and washing of hair after treatment.
 Special precautions necessary to protect the eyes.
 The keeping of inflammable preparations away from any
 source of naked flame.
N.B. Care should be taken with disposal of cotton wool mops, clean-
 ing of all equipment after use and treatment of all infested linen
 (including gown worn by nurse).

3. Trolley for hair-washing in bed

A large basin.
A bath thermometer.
A small bowl with cotton wool for the ears (if desired).

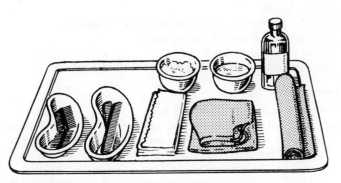

Figure 4.1
Tray for inspection of the hair and scalp

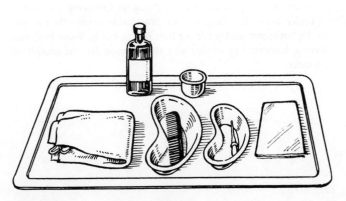

Figure 4.2
Tray for treatment of a verminous head

A face cloth in a receptacle.

A small jug or bottle with the shampoo. A special preparation, e.g. 'Derbac' or 'Esoderm', may be used following treatment of a verminous head or as a prophylactic measure.

A large jug of rinsing water.

A dressing comb.

A waterproof pillowcase.

A plastic shoulder cape.

Two bath towels.

Waterproof protection for the bed and floor as required.

A large jug with supply of rinsing water.

A bucket for soiled water.

A hair dryer may be used to complete the drying process.

Clinical notes

When the hair must be washed in bed:

Position the bed away from the wall and remove the bed head when possible or alternatively pull the mattress away from the head of the bed. Protect the patient, bed and floor. Place the basin on a chair or on the exposed end of the bed spring. Have the patient in the most comfortable position with head, neck and shoulders well supported.

Shampoo hair in the usual way, rinsing well. Dry thoroughly with a warm bath towel and hair dryer if available. Dress hair in a suitable manner.

Ensure warmth and protection from draughts following treatment.

This is undertaken only when it is not practicable to take the patient to the bathroom and wash the hair over a basin. Some hospitals have a hairdressing service and this is good for the morale of patients.

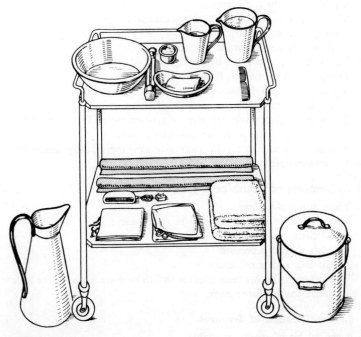

Figure 4.3
Trolley for hair-washing in bed

Care of mouth and teeth

1. Tray for cleaning the mouth

A disposable drape.

A polythene square for extra protection when necessary.

A mouthwash in a tumbler or a disposable cup.

A receptacle for the return wash.

Bottles containing the requisite lotions:

 Soda bicarbonate solution 1:160.

 Glycothymoline 1:10 (or one mouth wash tablet dissolved in half a tumbler of warm water).

 Glycerine (to which a little lemon juice may be added).

Three small gallipots.

A labelled denture container.

A receptacle with white cotton wool mops.

A receptacle with gauze swabs.

Disposal bag for discarded materials.

Lip salve to prevent lips becoming dry and cracked.

The patient's own tooth brush and paste.

A receptacle with disposable clamping forceps, wooden probes and tongue depressor.

A disposable glove when necessary, e.g. when caring for the mouth of a young infant or an unconscious patient.

Alternatively, and in certain circumstances, individually wrapped mouth care packs may be used.

2. Contents of mouth care pack

Three integral gallipots.

Polyether foam sponges secured to paper sticks.

Small tissues for use after swabbing.

Wooden tongue depressor.

Plastic bag and wire closure.

The lotions and other requisites for mouth care are added to the tray with the prepared pack.

3. Identification of dentures

A special kit is usually available.

Small abrasive pads.

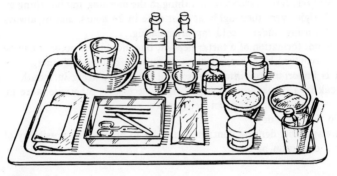

Figure 5.1
Tray for attention to mouth toilet

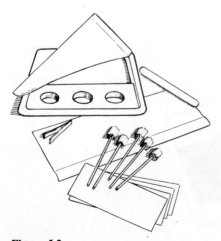

Figure 5.2
Individual mouth-care pack

A marking pencil.

A bottle of sealing liquid complete with applicator brush in the cap.

This is undertaken only when absolutely necessary but is particularly helpful in geriatric and psycho-geriatric wards.

4. General care of dentures

A suitable denture brush and ordinary soap and water may suffice.

Clean regularly: especially first thing in the morning and last thing at night, very thoroughly at least once in 24 hours, and by always rinsing under a cold tap after eating.

Prevent formation of a tartar deposit, but should this occur it can be removed by the application of an acid brush-on cleaner.

It is important to rinse denture well before replacing in mouth.

Soak in a hypochlorite solution when necessary, otherwise store in plain water when not being worn.

Do not store dry.

Always label denture container in order to obviate the possibility of confusion or loss.

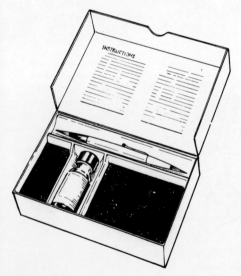

Figure 5.3
Denture identification kit

Notes

Administration of medicines (orally)

Mobile locking medicine trolley for storage of drugs in daily use:
An internal locking compartment for schedule poisons which have
    been prescribed.
Racks for small medicine bottles and containers.
Storage space for larger medicine bottles.
Small tray for taking drugs to the patient.
Jug of drinking water (milk may sometimes be required).
Graduated medicine glasses in holder.
Drinking straws and graduated spoons.
A box of tissues.
Disposal bag clipped to rail of trolley.
Kardex with patient's prescription sheets.
Pull out writing/dispensing tray.
Container for used glasses and spoons.
N.B. When in use the trolley should never be left unattended at any
    time.
When not in use the trolley should be locked and secured by padlock
    or other means to a *fixed point* on the wall or floor.
Safe custody of keys must be ensured at all times.

General guide for administration

Read the prescription carefully.
Ascertain that prescribed dose has not already been administered.
Select drug required and check the label with the prescription.
Prepare the drug in the presence of a witness who must have had the
    requisite training to enable him/her to check medicines as
    follows:
    The drug.
    The calculation, if any.
    The measured dose.
    The name of the patient.
Take the measured dose and prescription to the bedside, check identi-
    ty of the patient (with identiband when appropriate) and ad-
    minister the drug in the presence of the witness.

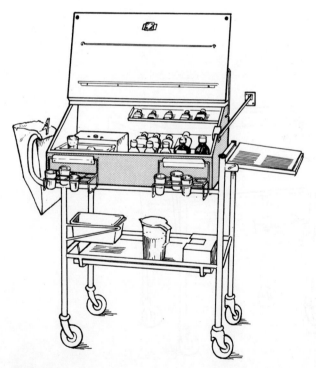

Figure 6.1
Mobile medicine trolley

N.B. Nurse must see the patient take the drug. Every dose of medicine administered should be recorded immediately on the appropriate recording sheet.

When a 'controlled drug' has been given, the relevant details should be entered in the 'Controlled Drugs Register'.

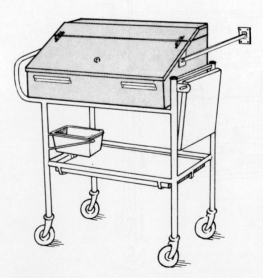

Figure 6.2
Medicine trolley – locked and secured to a fixed point

Notes

Metric system of weights and measures

The current version is known as *Système International d'Unités* (SI units)

There are seven basic units.

		Symbol
Length	metre	m
Mass	kilogram	kg
Time	second	s
Electric current	ampere	A
Temperature	kelvin	K
Luminous intensity	candela	cd
Amount of substance	mole	mol

The SI unit of volume is the cubic metre but the litre is accepted and defined as exactly equivalent to one cubic decimetre, i.e.

    1 litre = 1 cubic decimetre

    1000 litres = 1 cubic metre

All other multiples and sub-multiples are derived from these basic units.

Decimal multiples and sub-multiples are expressed as follows:

Multiplication factor		Prefix	Symbol
1 000 000	10^{6}	mega	M
1 000	10^{3}	kilo	k
0.1	10^{-1}	deci	d
0.01	10^{-2}	centi	c
0.001	10^{-3}	milli	m
0.000 001	10^{-6}	micro	μ

Nurses will commonly use four of the basic units:

    metre; kilogram; second; mole.

Also the *litre* for measuring volume and the *kilojoule* (kJ) used for measuring the heat and energy value of food.

Useful tables

1. Mass

10 milligrams = 1 centigram
10 centigrams = 1 decigram
10 decigrams = 1 gram
10 grams = 1 decagram
10 decagrams = 1 hectagram
10 hectagrams = 1 kilogram

The *milligram*, the *gram* and the *kilogram* are the units in most common use.

The *microgram*, which is 1/1000 part of a milligram is used when very small doses are required.

For quantities less than 1 gram it is recommended that drugs be prescribed in milligrams or micrograms whichever is appropriate.

This avoids the use of the decimal point, as a whole number minimises the danger of confusion or error.

For example: 0.5 gram = 500 milligrams

To convert grams to milligrams move the decimal point three places to the right.

When the decimal point is used it must never stand 'naked', e.g. .5, but must have a zero in front, 0.5.

2. Volume

10 millilitres = 1 centilitre
10 centilitres = 1 decilitre
10 decilitres = 1 litre

Only two units are in common use:
the *millilitre* and the *litre*
1000 millilitres = 1 litre

The symbol for a unit is unaltered in the plural and should not be followed by a full stop unless at the close of a sentence, e.g. 100 ml or 5 cm, *not* 100 ml. or 5 cms.

Notes

Equipment for recording body temperature

Clinical thermometers

These are calibrated glass tubes containing mercury. Each patient has an individual thermometer.

Types:

Standard. Registering 35°C to 43.5°C.

Low registering. Records down to 21°C.

Rectal. Distinctive features are a short, blunt bulb for ease of insertion and coloured bulb for identification purposes.

Temtake

Temperature taker which is a single use thermometer.

Features: A combination of chemicals contained in small cavities in an aluminium strip. The recording head is sealed under a plastic layer and gives a temperature reading to 0.1°C or 0.2°F.

The celsius version gives readings from 35.5°C to 40.4°C.

Oral temperature can be recorded accurately in 60 seconds. It may also be used in the axilla or groin but recording time is three minutes and it should be taped in position. Irradiation following manufacture ensures freedom from micro-organisms.

Being discarded after use minimises risk of 'cross infection'.

Electronic thermometer

This may be used in certain circumstances.

Features include: Simple press button which gives maximum temperature measurement in a few seconds (range 32°C to 42°C).

Choice of thermister sensor probes;

Rigid, glass tipped for oral or armpit use.

Flexible plastic, with suitable length of cord for rectal use.

Other requisites

Cotton wool mops for drying skin surfaces and wiping clinical thermometers.

A lubricant for rectal thermometers.

Disposal bag.

Watch with seconds hand.

Pen or pencil and chart or Kardex.

N.B. Ensure that clinical thermometers are cleaned and re-set after use. They must also be disinfected as required.

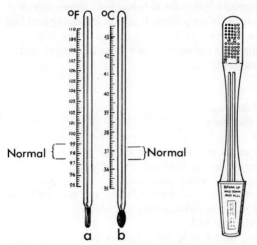

Normal { }

} Normal

a   b

Figure 7.1

Figure 7.2

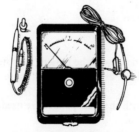

Figure 7.3

Figure 7.1
Clinical thermometer a. oral bulb, Fahrenheit scale b. rectal bulb, Celsius scale

Figure 7.2
Temtake – single use temperature taker

Figure 7.3
Electronic thermometer

Tepid sponging

This treatment is carried out in order to reduce body temperature and improve the comfort of the patient. It aims at increasing heat loss by evaporation of moisture from the surface of the skin.

It is not usual to attempt a reduction of more than one degree celsius during the treatment.

Requirements

Trolley with the following:
A large basin for the water.
Bath thermometer.
A bowl with six sponges or soft washing cloths.
Bowl with two compresses for forehead, in iced water.
Clinical thermometer and cotton wool swabs.
Two large jugs, one with tepid water (26°C), and one with cold water to cool water in basin during procedure.
Waterproof protection for bed.
Two bathing sheets, bath towels and a face cloth.
Clean gown and bed linen.
Bucket for used water.
Receptacle for soiled linen.

Clinical notes

If water which is too cold is used, the patient may start to shiver and this should be avoided as shivering will raise the body temperature.

Long sweeping strokes with the wet sponges are used, leaving beads of moisture on the skin.

Wet sponges are placed in the axillae and groins and changed at intervals.

The compress on the forehead is also changed frequently.

Temperature is recorded before and after treatment which takes 15 to 20 minutes. Should the patient suffer any untoward effects or the temperature fall sharply, the treatment should be stopped immediately. The patient is kept under observation and temperature again recorded 30 minutes after treatment. It usually continues to fall slowly. Patient is left dry and comfortable, what light clothing as is allowed should be replaced.

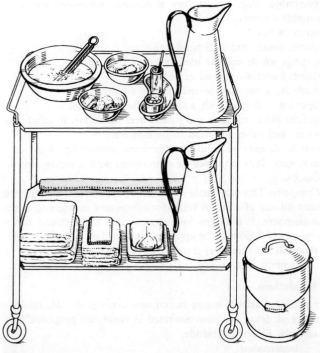

Figure 8
Trolley for tepid sponging

Inhalations

Tray for medicated steam inhalation

An earthenware inhaler (Nelson's).

A bowl in which to stand the inhaler.

A flannel bag to cover the inhaler (air inlet always exposed).

A glass mouthpiece and a gauze swab to wrap round it to protect the lips.

A graduated jug with 550ml of water, temperature 71°C.

The water level in the inhaler must always be below the level of the air inlet.

A lotion thermometer.

The prescribed drug, e.g. tincture of benzoin compound, and a suitable measure.

A sputum carton.

Disposable tissues and a disposal bag.

Other drugs which may be used include:

Menthol crystals and oil of eucalyptus.

Alternatively, a jug may be used as the inhaler.

The opening is draped with a towel to form a funnel.

The patient places his nose and mouth over the funnel to inhale the steam and raises his head to breathe out.

A steam kettle may be used for continuous moistening of the atmosphere. It is employed in conjunction with a steam tent canopy.

The Croupaire. This is a simple and effective apparatus which may be used instead of a steam kettle for continuous moistening of the atmosphere. It is driven by electricity and the reservoir has a capacity of 3000 ml. The apparatus is placed on a locker or table about 60 to 65 cm away from the patient's face. A fine stream of cool vapour mist is directed towards the patient.

Dry inhalations

The pressurised aerosol is now in common use, e.g. the 'Medihaler'.

A number of drugs are now marketed in these 'self-propelled' aerosols. Examples include:

Isoprenaline.

Adrenaline.

Phenylephrine.

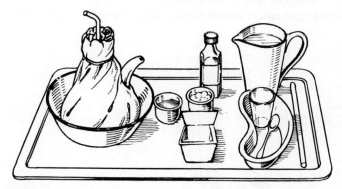

Figure 9.1
Tray for medicated steam inhalation

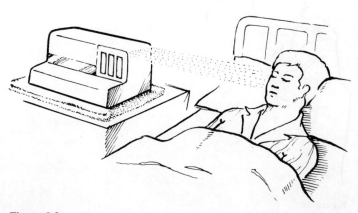

Figure 9.2
Croupaire

These preparations are ordered for relief of bronchospasm.

A metered dose of the drug is delivered each time the valve is released.

Instructions on how to use the inhaler are provided by the manufacturer and great care must be taken to *ensure that the prescribed dose is not exceeded.*

Dangers of misuse and overdosage should be clearly understood.

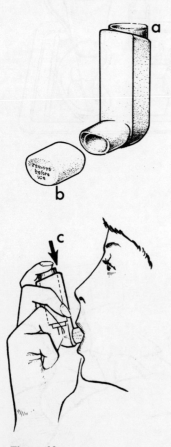

Figure 10
Medihaler a. drug container b. dust cover c. inspiration and pressure on vial should be synchronised

Notes

Oxygen therapy

Requirements

A source of oxygen supply which may be a cylinder on a mobile stand or a 'pipe line' to a fixed oxygen point on the wall beside the patient's bed.

A pressure reducing gauge and flowmeter.

A humidifier filled to the appropriate level with distilled water. A variety of designs are available.

Pressure tubing of suitable length to connect the source of the oxygen to the apparatus being used for administration, and a glass connection when necessary.

Examples of apparatus

1. *The Ventimask* which is designed to enable a low concentration of oxygen to be given. Three models are available and with the rate of flow adjusted according to instructions they will deliver 24, 28 and 35 per cent oxygen respectively.

2. *The Edinburgh mask* is similar in principle to the Ventimask and also enables a low concentration of oxygen to be given. A flow rate of 4 to 6 litres per minute will provide 23 to 35 per cent inspired oxygen concentration.

N.B. When carefully controlled, low concentration oxygen therapy is essential as in, for example, chronic bronchitis, the correct choice of mask is of the utmost importance if carbon dioxide narcosis and underventilation is to be avoided.

3. *The Polymask.*

4. *M C mask.* (3) and (4) will deliver a much higher concentration of oxygen, 40 to 60 per cent with a flow rate of 6 to 8 litres per minute.

5. *Nasal catheters.* The type most commonly used is the double cannulae with a Y connection for attachment to pressure tubing. With a flow rate of 2 litres per minute the inspired oxygen concentration may be raised to 30 per cent but this is unpredictable and less easily controlled. A small tray with requisites for cleaning the nostrils should be available.

6. *Oxygen tents.* A variety of designs are available to suit both infants and adults. The maker's instructions should always be

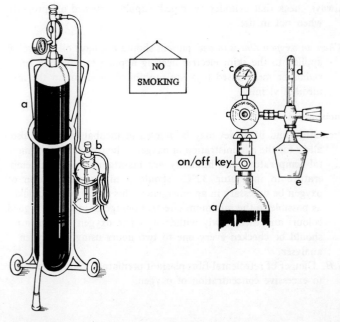

NO SMOKING

on/off key

Figure 11.1
a. oxygen cylinder b. humidifier/flowmeter c. gauge d. flowmeter e. nebuliser

followed carefully to ensure satisfactory operation of the equipment.

Clinical notes

Oxygen therapy is prescribed very frequently and instructions should be in writing regarding apparatus to be used, rate of flow and concentration required.

Dangers of fire

Ensure adequate instruction of all staff; supervision of patients and visitors; 'No Smoking' notices clearly displayed; no matches, cigarettes, lighters or naked flames of any kind in the vicinity of the oxygen.

Continuous observation of patient's condition.

Equipment checked regularly and properly maintained. No oils or grease used on taps or valves.

Cylinders should be handled with care and stored in a cool place.

Always check that cylinder or 'piped' supply is turned off properly when not in use.

When an oxygen tent is in use, patient should not have oil or alcohol applied to the skin; electric heating appliances, shavers, bells, radios or mechanised toys are prohibited inside or in the immediate vicinity.

Incubators

Premature and ill babies may be nursed in incubators which also allow for the administration of oxygen. The correct environmental temperature and humidity are maintained (average temperature in incubator 32°C). Should a high concentration of oxygen be necessary in an emergency, this is reduced as quickly as possible to the minimum effective dosage to maintain a good colour, and then slowly withdrawn. The oxygen concentration should be checked every one to two hours using an oxygen analyser.

N.B. Danger of retrolental fibroplasia if premature infant is exposed to excessive concentration of oxygen.

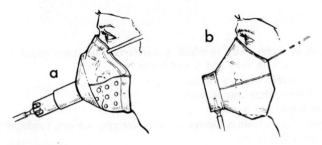

Figure 11.2
a. Ventimask
b. Edinburgh mask

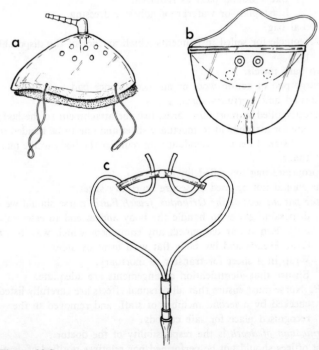

Figure 11.3
a. MC mask b. Polymask c. Nasal cannula (Argyle)

Trolley for last offices to the dead

A basin of warm water to which a disinfectant has been added.

A receptacle with soap and a nail brush.

Two disposable washing cloths.

A bowl with white cotton wool.

A hair brush and comb.

A small tray with sinus forceps, dressing forceps, scissors, bandages and a roll of tape.

When there is a dressing add:

> A suitable sized dressing pack.
> Disinfectant solution.
> Extra wound pads as required.
> Elastoplast or waterproof adhesive dressing.

Disposal bag.

A receptacle for soiled instruments which are not of the disposable type.

Two bath towels.

A large pad of cotton wool or an incontinence pad.

A shroud and mortuary sheet.

Correctly filled in mortuary cards, two for attachment to the body, one for attachment to mortuary sheet and one to be handed to, and signed by, the attendant who removes the body to the mortuary.

Appropriate bag for soiled linen.

Pins should not be used to secure mortuary sheet.

If the patient was of the Orthodox Jewish Faith, nurse should wear disposable gloves to handle the body and attend to essentials only: Remove or disconnect any equipment which was in use.

Close eyelids and lay body flat with arms by sides.

Wrap in a sheet for transfer to mortuary.

Ensure that identification arrangements are adequate.

N.B. Nurse must ensure that all personal effects are carefully listed, checked by a second member of staff, and removed to the recognised place for safe custody.

Verification of death is the responsibility of the doctor.

Last offices should not be performed nor relatives notified of death until this has been done.

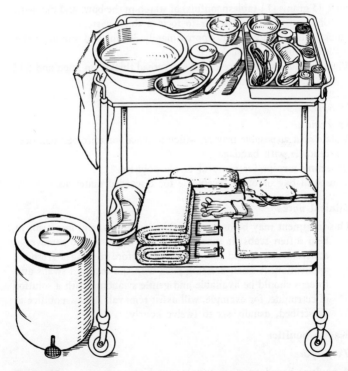

Figure 12
Trolley for last offices

Local applications

Starch poultice

To prepare

A poultice board or other suitable working surface.

A jar with starch powder.

A jug with cold water.

A kettle with boiling water.

A large bowl.

A tablespoon, a wooden spoon and a spatula.

A suitable sized piece of old linen.

Place 45 grams ($1\frac{1}{2}$ tablespoonfuls) of starch in the bowl and mix with only sufficient cold water to form a thick paste.

Quickly add boiling water, approximately 300 ml and stir until the starch begins to thicken.

When poultice is almost cold and set, spread thickly on linen and fold in margins smoothly.

To apply

Tray with:

A plate or a disposable tray on which to place the unfolded poultice.

A receptacle with bandage.

Dissecting forceps for removal of old poultice.

A disposal bag or other receptacle for discarded materials.

Clinical notes

This treatment may be ordered in skin conditions, e.g. impetigo, to help soften scabs. It may therefore be necessary to remove adherent starch and loosened crusts before making a fresh application. A small dressing pack with the required swabs and forceps should be available and gentle swabbing with a solution of cetrimide, for example, will assist removal. Renew poultice as prescribed, usually six to twelve hourly.

Kaolin poultice

To prepare

A poultice board or other suitable working surface.

A tin of kaolin (lid removed and contents well stirred).

A small pan in which to heat the kaolin (pan half filled with boiling
   water).
A spatula.
A suitably sized piece of old linen and a layer of gauze.
Heat the kaolin by allowing the tin to simmer in boiling water for 10
   to 15 minutes. Stir the contents well. Remove tin from pan, place
   on working surface, spread kaolin evenly on linen with spatula,
   cover surface with a layer of gauze and fold in margins smoothly.

To apply

Tray with:
Prepared poultice between two well heated plates.
A receptacle with a piece of cotton wool to cover the poultice, a bandage or binder, and safety pins.
For skin care between applications or on completion of treatment add
   the following:
      A bottle of olive oil and a gallipot.
      Cotton wool mops.
      A receptacle for soiled mops.
N.B. Ensure that discarded poultice is placed with soiled dressings
   for disposal and not with soiled linen for the laundry. Kaolin
   presents a grave fire hazard if put in a tumbler dryer.

Clinical notes

This treatment may be ordered for relief of pain in pleurisy,
   pneumonia and the early stages of local inflammation.
The heat of the poultice should be tested on the back of nurse's hand
   to prevent danger of burning the patient. Repeat application
   as prescribed, e.g. four to six hourly.

Tray for application of a cold compress

Two bowls – one with cold water and one with pieces of ice.
Several single layers of old linen or lint in a receptacle.
A receptacle in which to place compress on removal.
A disposable towel and waterproof protection.
A bottle of eau de Cologne if being applied for relief of headache.
A bed cradle may be required to permit the evaporation necessary to
   keep the part cool.

An ice bag

To prepare

A poultice board or other suitable working surface.
A bowl with chopped ice.
A bowl with tepid water (in which to swill the sharp edges off the ice).
A jar of salt, and a teaspoon.
An ice pick.
A flannel square on which to chop ice.
An ice bag, or a polythene bag and cellotape to seal the end.
A towel to dry the bag.

To apply

Tray with:
The ice bag in a cover.
A receptacle with a bandage and safety pins.
(A bed cradle may be required from which to suspend the bag).
Proprietary packs of 'dry ice' may be used for the application of cold.
    Follow manufacturer's instructions.

Clinical notes

Cold applications may be prescribed for:
Limitation of effusion following injury, e.g. to a joint; early treatment
    of inflammation of non-bacterial origin; control of haemorrhage;
    relief of pain.
N.B. Dangers of prolonged application of cold include:
    Pain.
    Redness.
    Mottling of the skin.
    'Ice-burn'.

Enemas

Administration of an evacuant enema

1. *Disposable unit*

The disposable enema unit containing 120 ml of a solution of sodium phosphate.

A diposable rectal catheter may be added when necessary although some units have a long tube attached.

A bowl with warm water in which to heat the unit.

The solution may be given at room temperature.

Catheter lubricating jelly.

A gallipot with cotton wool mops.

A disposal bag.

Polythene and disposable drape or an incontinence pad.

A warmed bed pan and disposable cover.

2. *'Tube and funnel' method*

A rectal catheter, size 12, a connection and length of tubing, a funnel, and tubing clamp.

A soap solution. This is prepared in a graduated jug and kept at a suitable temperature (37.7°C). Usual volume for an adult 600 to 1000 ml.

Other requisites as in (1) above.

Although still in use, many authorities consider this method to be obsolete.

Care must be taken with subsequent cleaning of any apparatus which is not disposable.

3. *'Micralax' enema*

The disposable unit containing 5 ml of a solution of sodium and sorbic acid. It is used when only a small volume of solution is indicated, e.g. in dyschezia or prior to proctoscopy.

Other requisites as in (1).

It is not necessary to warm the unit.

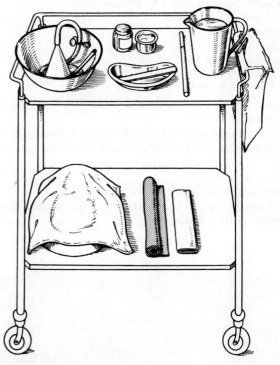

Figure 13.1
Trolley for an evacuant enema

4. *Other solutions which may be used and are available in disposable units*

Arachis or olive oil 130 ml. This is given to soften hard or impacted faeces.

Magnesium sulphate 25 per cent solution. This is hygroscopic, produces a watery stool and may be used as an adjunct to neurosurgery.

Administration of a retention enema

1. *Disposable enema unit*

The enema unit containing the solution to be administered, e.g. solution of prednisolone which is used in the local treatment of ulcerative colitis.

A bowl with warm water in which to heat the unit.

A gallipot with cotton wool mops.

Catheter lubricating jelly.

A disposal bag.

Suitable protection for the bed.

2. *'Tube and funnel' method*

A rectal catheter, size 8, a connection and length of tubing, and a cylindrical funnel.

A graduated jug with the solution to be administered standing in a bowl of warm water. (A 5 per cent glucose saline solution may be given rectally in fluid replacement therapy).

Other requisites as in (1).

Fluids for retention should be introduced slowly.

A bed elevator may be required to raise the foot of the bed and thus aid retention of the solution.

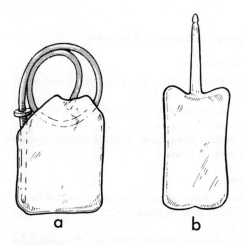

Figure 13.2
Disposable enema units   a. long tube   b. standard

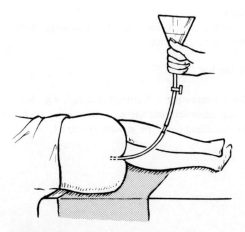

Figure 13.3
Position for administration of an enema

Suppositories

There are two main groups, *evacuant* and *retention*.

Evacuant types in common use

Glycerin (solidified with gelatin). This acts as a hygroscopic agent and stimulates evacuation of the bowel.

Bisacodyl (Dulcolax). This increases the secretion of the mucous membranes in the lower bowel and thus aids evacuation.

Beogex. A proprietary sodium preparation which stimulates evacuation by liberating carbon dioxide.

Retention suppositories

Prednisolone. Prescribed as local treatment in ulcerative colitis.

Aminophylline. Prescribed in an appropriate dosage for the treatment of bronchial spasm.

Pentazocine (Fortral) or dextromoramide (Palfium). Prescribed for their analgesic effect.

Requisites for administration

Small tray with:

The prescribed suppository.

Lubricating jelly, except in the case of 'Beogex' when the suppository should be moistened in plain water.

Disposable glove.

Appropriate protection for bed.

Disposal bag.

N.B. When a suppository containing a 'controlled drug', e.g. dextromoramide, is being administered, the code of practice regarding checking and recording must be strictly observed.

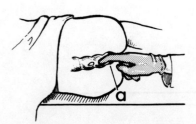

Figure 14
Insertion of a suppository beyond the internal anal sphincter (a)

Flatus tube

This is a rectal tube which is passed for relief of abdominal distension.

Requisites

Tray with:

Disposable flatus tube and when required an extra length of tubing and a glass connection.

A bowl of warm water to which an antiseptic has been added.

Other requisites for lubricating tube, cleansing the anal region and protection of the bed.

Disposal bag.

N.B. Before the introduction of any rectal tubes or suppositories the patient should be given an adequate explanation of the treatment and also be provided with facilities for emptying the bladder.

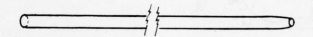

Figure 15
Flatus tube

Rectal examination

This may be carried out by the digital method only or by use of a proctoscope which may or may not be electrically illuminated.

Indications for such an examination

Haemorrhoids.
Suspected new growths of the rectum, e.g. carcinoma.
Anal fistula.
Pelvic conditions such as pelvic abscess.
Disease of the reproductive organs.
Prostatic enlargement.

Requirements

Tray or trolley with the following:
Disposable drape.
Receptacle with disposable examination gloves.
Container with finger cots.
Receptacle with gauze swabs.
Lubricating jelly.
Receptacle with proctoscope which may be of the disposable variety or the electrically illuminated type.
A specimen container when necessary.
Disposal bag for used gloves, swabs and finger cots.
Disposable towel on which to place used instruments.
A good light should be available.

Clinical notes

The examination may include the sigmoid colon, when an illuminated sigmoidoscope would be used.
Always check the bulbs in equipment before use.
Doctor may, in certain circumstances, order special preparation such as a plain water enema on the evening before examination.
Patient may be placed in the left lateral or knee chest position with adequate protection being provided.

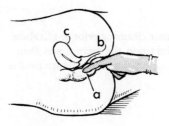

Figure 16.1
Digital examination of the rectum   a. finger in rectum   b. the vaginal canal
 c. the uterus

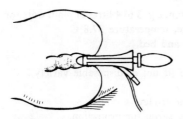

Figure 16.2
Visual rectal examination – using an illuminated proctoscope

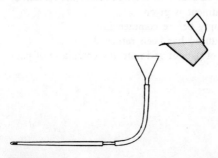

Figure 16.3
Barium enema – preparation for X-ray examination

Rectal lavage (wash-out)

This may be ordered to ensure adequate cleansing prior to rectal surgery. It involves introducing fluid into the rectum and then siphoning it back again. This is repeated until the return fluid is as clear as possible.

Requirements

Trolley with the following:

A large bowl with the apparatus – a funnel, length of tubing, glass connection, rectal tube and clip.

Lubricant and a gallipot with cotton wool mops.

Lotion thermometer.

A measuring jug (600 ml capacity).

A large jug with the wash-out lotion, e.g. 3 to 4 litres of plain water or solution of soda bicarbonate, temperature 37.8°C.

Waterproof protection for floor and bed.

Disposable drape.

Receptacle for soiled rectal tube (if not of disposable variety).

A bucket for the return wash.

A disposal bag is attached to the trolley.

Nurse wears a disposable plastic apron for protection.

Clinical notes

Position and preparation of patient as for an enema.

It may be necessary to give an evacuant enema to clear the rectum of faeces before the treatment is given.

Ensure that bladder is empty before commencing.

Check that all fluid introduced has been returned.

Observe general condition of patient and note any complaint of pain or discomfort.

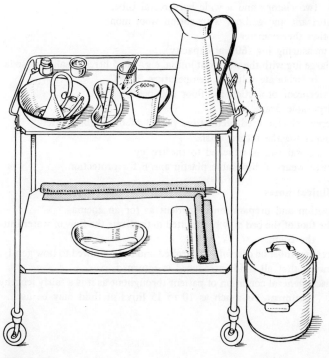

Figure 17
Trolley for rectal lavage

Colonic lavage (irrigation)

Indications for this treatment include:

Preparation for large bowel surgery, when it is carried out daily for a few days before the operation.

Prior to some X-ray examination of the colon.

As a therapeutic measure in diverticulosis.

Requirements

Trolley with the following:

A large bowl with a graduated irrigation can (a funnel may be used).

Receptacle with two lengths of tubing, a Y-shaped glass connection, two clamps and a wide bore rectal tube.

Lubricant and gallipot with cotton wool mops.

Lotion thermometer.

A measuring jug (600 ml capacity).

A large jug with the wash-out lotion, e.g. 4 to 5 litres of saline or soda bicarbonate solution, temperature 37.8°C.

Waterproof protection for floor and bed.

Disposable drape.

Receptacle for used rectal tube (if not of disposable variety).

Bucket for the return wash.

A disposal bag is attached to the trolley.

Nurse wears a disposable plastic apron for protection.

Clinical notes

Position and preparation of patient as for an enema.

The foot of the bed may be elevated to facilitate the flow of water into the colon.

Pressure must be carefully controlled and fluid allowed to flow gently.

Ensure that all fluid introduced is returned.

Assess general condition of patient throughout as it is a fairly lengthy treatment. As much as 10 to 15 litres of fluid may be used.

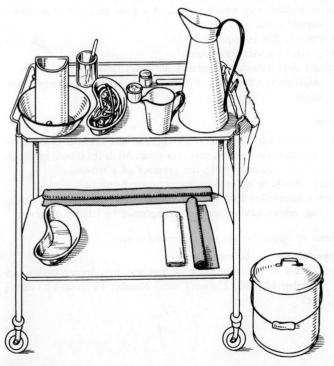

Figure 18
Trolley for colonic lavage

Injections

When it is necessary to administer drugs parenterally ('para' – outside, 'enteron' – the bowel), one of the following injection methods may be chosen.

Hypodermic (Subcutaneous). *Intramuscular. Intravenous.*

Basic equipment

Sterile syringe and needle(s) of suitable size.

Sterile disposable tray on which to take the charged syringe to the patient.

Sterile swabs impregnated with a skin disinfectant.

The prescribed drug which may be in a glass ampoule or a rubber capped bottle.

An ampoule file as required.

The patient's prescription sheet.

A single dose automatic injection unit may be available for administering some drugs by the subcutaneous or intramuscular route.

Notes

Strict asepsis must be observed and great care taken to avoid contamination of syringe, needle or drug. All drugs should be checked and administered in the presence of a witness.

Details should be entered in the patient's Kardex.

When a 'controlled drug' is given, the hospital rules regarding checking, administration and recording must be strictly observed.

Choice of apparatus for the prescribed route:

Hypodermic, i.e. beneath the skin

Usually a 1 or 2 ml disposable syringe and hypodermic needle e.g. Number 12 (23G) 25 mm (1 inch). Number 18 (26G) 15.5 mm ($\frac{5}{8}$ inch).

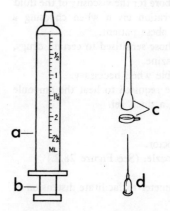

Figure 19.1
Hypodermic syringe   a. barrel   b. piston   c. needle cover and seal   d. needle

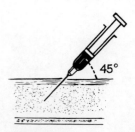

Figure 19.2
Hypodermic injection technique

Intramuscular, i.e. into a muscle

Usually a 2 or 5 ml disposable syringe although a larger one may sometimes be necessary.

Intramuscular or serum needles. These should be at least 50.5mm (2 inches) in length and of suitable bore for the viscosity of the fluid to be injected. Careful consideration given when choosing a needle for a very emaciated or obese patient.

Gloves may require to be worn by those sensitised to certain drugs, e.g. streptomycin or chlorpromazine.

A disposable mask should be available when necessary.

A small bowl of warm water may be required to heat the ampoule containing a drug which forms a thick gel.

Intravenous, i.e. into a vein

This is normally performed by a doctor.

5 or 10 ml syringe with eccentric nozzle. (See Figure 28.2.)

Intravenous needles.

Rubber tourniquet or sphygmomanometer to facilitate distension of the vein.

When specimens of blood are required, the appropriate tubes are added to the tray with requisites for venepuncture.

Other injection routes

Intradermal, i.e. into the skin itself, used for diagnostic purposes such as testing for sensitivity and also in commencement of local anaesthesia.

Intrathecal, i.e. when a drug is injected into the cerebro-spinal fluid, e.g. in the treatment of meningitis.

Intra-articular, e.g. when a drug is injected into an inflamed joint.

These techniques are always carried out by the doctor.

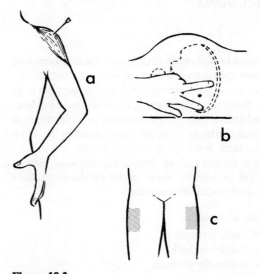

Figure 19.3
Sites chosen for intramuscular injections a. deltoid b. the anterior gluteal
(the index finger is placed on the anterior superior iliac spine and the middle
finger just below the iliac crest) c. anterolateral aspect of the thigh

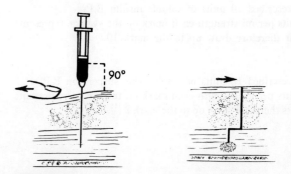

Figure 19.4
Intramuscular injection technique and the skin back in place after
withdrawal of the needle

Insulin injections

A special insulin syringe is used which is calibrated for measurements in units, although the term units does not appear on the syringe. A 1 ml syringe has twenty divisions and a 2 ml syringe has forty divisions, thus facilitating the drawing up of an accurate dose.

Doses are calculated individually for each patient and prescribed in units. The insulin may be injected hypodermically or intramuscularly, the same route being used each time.

N.B. In emergency situations such as diabetic keto-acidosis (diabetic coma) doctor will usually give some insulin by the intravenous route in the initial stages of treatment.

Standard strengths of insulin

20 units per ml or single strength.
40 units per ml or double strength.
80 units per ml or quadruple strength.

Each mark on an insulin syringe represents:

One unit if using 20 units per ml strength.
Two units if using 40 units per ml strength.
Four units if using 80 units per ml strength.

Example 1

Patient is prescribed 10 units of soluble insulin B.P.

Using 20 units per ml strength each mark on the syringe represents one unit therefore draw up to the mark 10.

Example 2

Patient is prescribed 16 units of insulin zinc suspension B.P.

Using 40 units per ml strength each mark on the syringe represents two units therefore draw up to the mark 8 $(\frac{16}{2} = 8)$.

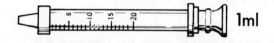

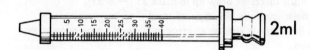

Figure 20.1
Insulin syringes

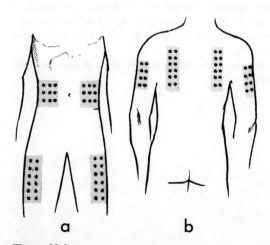

Figure 20.2
Rotation of sites for injection of insulin   a. anterior – may be self administered   b. posterior – alternatives

Example 3

Patient is prescribed 48 units of insulin zinc suspension B.P. (crystalline).

Using 80 units per ml strength each mark on the syringe represents four units therefore draw up to the mark 12 ($\frac{48}{4} = 12$).

For over 80 units a 2 ml syringe is necessary.

Example 4

Patient is prescribed 92 units of insulin zinc suspension B.P. (amorphous).

Using 80 units per ml strength each mark on the syringe represents four units therefore draw up to mark 23 ($\frac{92}{4} = 23$).

Always check carefully the type of insulin to be given.

Accuracy in dosage is vital as an error may cause a patient to go into a coma.

Dose should be checked by a second person.

Record each dose on patient's insulin record chart.

If a combination of soluble insulin and protamine zinc insulin has been prescribed always confirm the method of preparing the injection. Some physicians will advise that the two insulins should never be mixed in the same syringe but may be given via the same injection puncture. Should it be considered permissible to give both types of insulin in one syringe, the soluble insulin should be drawn up first, followed by the P.Z.I. and the injection given immediately.

Rotation of injection sites is important in prevention of tissue atrophy or hypertrophy.

Artificial feeding

Methods by which food may be introduced into the alimentary tract.

1. Intra-nasal or intra-oral oesophageal feeding

Requirements

A trolley which has been thoroughly washed and dried.

A graduated jug containing the feed at the correct temperature (37.7°C), standing in a bowl of warm water.

Food thermometer.

A tray with the apparatus, i.e. a cylindrical funnel or 50 ml syringe, a suitable length of tubing, a glass connection, a gate clip and a disposable oesophageal tube or nasal catheter of appropriate size for an adult or child.

Container with a measured volume of water (sufficient to expel air from apparatus before the feed and clear the tube after the feed).

Lubricant, e.g. liquid paraffin or glycerine, and a gallipot.

10 ml syringe and litmus paper in a receptacle.

Bowl with gauze swabs.

Requisites for cleansing nostrils if intra-nasal route is used.

Receptacle with mouth gag, tongue forceps and spatula if the patient is unconscious or unable to co-operate.

A disposal bag.

Disposable drape and waterproof protection.

A sickness basin and tissues.

Receptacle with scissors, adhesive strapping and a spigot when necessary.

Clinical notes

Passing of oesophageal tube:

Conscious patient should be sitting up well supported.

Unconscious patient should be on his/her side to guard against inhalation of regurgitated feed (tube should be passed by doctor or qualified nurse).

Nasal tube is passed backwards along the floor of the nose into the pharynx, oesophagus and stomach. *Always check* that it does not curl forward into the mouth.

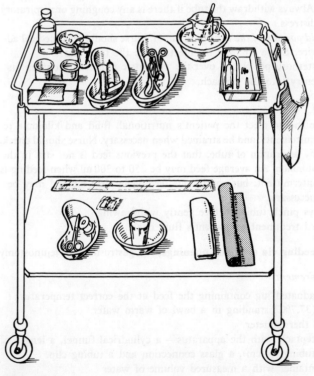

Figure 21.1
Trolley for intra-nasal or intra-oral oesophageal feeding

65

Oral tube is introduced at the side of the mouth and passed backward *avoiding the uvula*, patient being instructed to take deep breaths, and swallow as the tube is passed into the pharynx, oesophagus and stomach.

Checking that tube is in the stomach

Ensure that sufficient length of tube has been passed to reach the stomach, usually 50 cm in an adult.

Aspirate a small amount of fluid into syringe and test with litmus paper. If reaction is acid, tube is in stomach. If no fluid is withdrawn, the end of the tube may be placed under the surface of water in a bowl and escape of bubbles coinciding with expiration would indicate that it is in the air passage.

N.B. Always withdraw the tube if there is any coughing or respiratory distress.

Should position of the tube be in doubt, nurse should seek medical advice. Some air may be injected into the tube and a stethoscope placed over the epigastric region to confirm its entry into the stomach.

Feeds

These should meet the patient's nutritional, fluid and kilojoule requirements, and be strained when necessary. Nurse should check, by aspiration of tube, that the previous feed is not still in the stomach. An average feed may be 250 to 300 ml when feeding is intermittent, but continuous feeding by drip method may be necessary.

Always pinch tubing before gently withdrawing.

Record treatment on patient's fluid chart.

2. **Feeding via artificial openings,** e.g. gastrostomy or jejunostomy

Requirements

A graduated jug containing the feed at the correct temperature (37.7°C) standing in a bowl of warm water.

Food thermometer.

A receptacle with the apparatus – a cylindrical funnel, a length of tubing (30 cm), a glass connection and a tubing clip.

A container with a measured volume of water.

Gauze swabs and a dressing pad.

Scissors and adhesive tape to fix dressing in position.

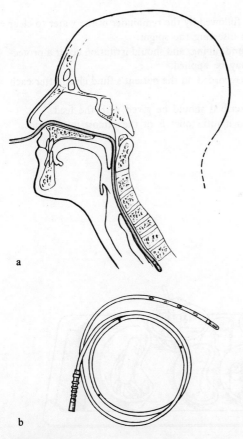

Figure 21.2
a. passing of a Ryle's tube   b. Ryle's tube

A disposable drape and waterproof protection.
Receptacle for discarded dressings.

Clinical notes

Kilojoule value and constituents of feed will vary with the needs of
the patient. Special feeds may be supplied from the diet kitchen.
Patient should be sitting up.
Nurse's hands washed thoroughly.
A little water should be allowed to run through the apparatus before
giving the feed.
Feed is given slowly, followed by the remainder of the water to clear
the tube, before inserting the spigot.
Attention to skin around tubing, and should irritation occur a protec-
tive ointment may be applied.
Treatment should be recorded on the patient's fluid chart after each
feed.
Oral medication prescribed should be given with the feed.
Frequent attention to mouth toilet is of the utmost importance.

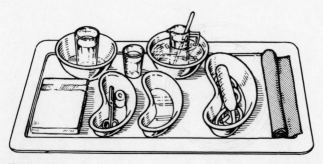

Figure 22.1
Tray for gastrostomy feeding

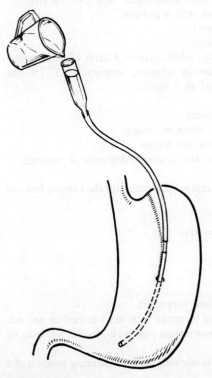

Figure 22.2
Introducing a gastrostomy feed – funnel tilted to allow escape of air

Gastric lavage (wash out)

Indications for treatment

Non-corrosive poisoning, e.g. barbiturate.

Pyloric stenosis.

Pre-operative treatment in certain cases of gastric surgery.

The need to procure specimens for examination.

Requirements on trolley

A large bowl with the apparatus – conical funnel, length of tubing, glass connection and large oesophageal tube (No. 18 EG).

Lubricant such as glycerine, and a gallipot.

Gauze swabs in a small bowl.

Receptacle with 20 ml syringe.

A large jug with the solution which may be 4 litres of plain water, saline, or soda bicarbonate solution, temperature 37.7°C (introduced usually 300 ml at a time).

Lotion thermometer.

Graduated jug, 1 litre capacity.

Labelled denture container when necessary.

A mouth wash and bowl for the return.

Receptacle with mouth gag and a tongue depressor if required.

Sickness basin and tissues.

A disposable drape and waterproof protection for the patient, bed and floor.

Bucket for return wash.

Specimen jar(s) when necessary.

A disposal bag.

Clinical notes

Position of patient:

If conscious – sitting up, well supported.

If unconscious – semi-prone or prone with head turned to one side (doctor or qualified nurse should pass tube), foot of bed may be elevated.

Similar precautions as previously indicated for checking position of a gastric tube.

Follow medical instructions with regard to obtaining specimens of the
first fluid recovered from the stomach.

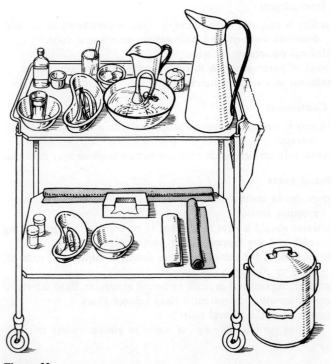

Figure 23
Trolley for gastric lavage

Gastric aspiration

This may be *intermittent* or *continuous*.

Indications for treatment

Pre-operatively in acute intestinal obstruction.

Post-operatively to rest the alimentary tract following gastrointestinal surgery.

In the non-operative treatment of obstruction due to paralytic ileus (paralysis of intestinal muscles).

To aspirate stomach contents for diagnostic purposes.

1. Intermittent

A trolley is prepared with the same basic requirements as already described for passing a naso-gastric oesophageal tube.

Additional equipment includes:

A bowl of water in which to rinse syringe between aspirations.

Graduated measure for aspirate.

2. Continuous

This may be carried out using a simple water flow arrangement as illustrated.

Alternatively, an electrically operated suction machine may be in use.

Clinical notes

Nurses should understand the principles involved in maintaining adequate suction.

Apparatus should always be checked to ensure that it is in working order and any blockage dealt with promptly.

The pressure of the suction machine should be adjusted as ordered, e.g. 5 to 10 mmHg.

Container emptied and aspirate measured at regular, fixed intervals.

Accurate recording on patient's fluid balance chart.

Frequent attention to oral toilet.

If condition permits, give sips of water or glucose sweets to suck.

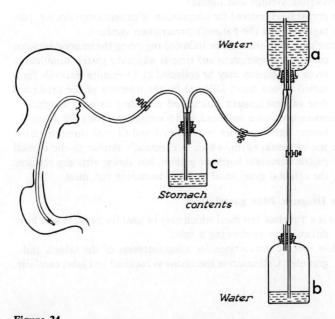

Figure 24

Wangensteen's apparatus for continuous gastric suction. Water flows from bottle 'a' to 'b' and a vacuum is created in bottle 'c' into which the stomach contents are aspirated

Fractional test meal

This treatment is ordered to enable the amount of acid in the stomach to be estimated and also to measure the amount of residual gastric contents after 12 hours fasting.

Requirements

Trolley with the basic equipment necessary for passing a Ryle's tube by the nasal or oral route, whichever is easier for the patient.

A measure for the fasting juice.

A rack with twelve numbered test tubes.

A bowl with water in which to rinse syringe after each specimen has been collected.

Hypodermic syringe and needle.

The preparation ordered for stimulation of gastric secretion, e.g. pentagastrin (on the patient's prescription card).

Doctor's instructions must be followed regarding the interval between collection of specimens and time at which the gastric stimulant is given. Specimens may be collected at 15 minute intervals for a period of one hour, followed by the injection of the prescribed dose of pentagastrin (calculated according to body weight).

Specimens are again collected at 15 minute intervals for $1\frac{1}{2}$ to 2 hours. Each specimen is measured and filtered through gauze.

The use of pentagastrin, which is chemically similar to the normal gastric stimulant hormone gastrin, has almost virtually replaced the original gruel meal and the histamine test meal.

The Diagnex Blue gastric test

This is a 'tubeless' test meal which may be used for patients who have difficulty in swallowing a tube.

Follow specific instructions for administration of the tablets and granules. Collect urine specimens as required and label carefully.

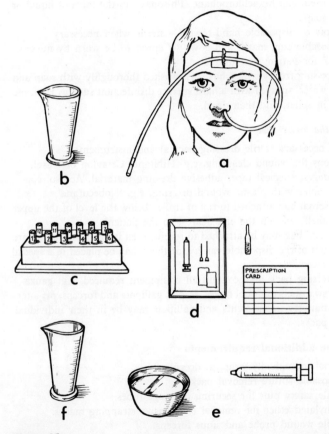

Figure 25
Fractional test meal a. Ryle's tube in position b. measure for fasting juice
c. numbered test tubes for specimens d. requisites for injection of the gastric
stimulant drug e. syringe and bowl with rinsing water f. measure for
residual juice

75

Preparation for surgical dressings

Basic equipment

Adequate facilities for hand washing. An antimicrobial agent may be
used, e.g. hexachlorophane (Phisohex), in the form of liquid or
soap.

Supply of disposable hand towels – sterile when necessary.

Disposable cap, mask, and gown or apron to be worn by nurse(s).
Mask for patient as required.

A dressing trolley which has been washed thoroughly with soap and
water, sprayed with a hard surface disinfectant such as Hibitane
in spirit, and then dried.

On the lower shelf

The necessary sterile dressing pack(s) and instruments.

Lotions for wound cleansing, e.g. Hibitane, Cetavlon or Eusol.

Bandages, surgical tape, adhesive dressing material. Aerosol container with plastic wound dressing, e.g. 'Nobecutane'.

A disposal bag attached to rail of trolley below the level of the upper
shelf, and on the end nearest to the patient.

A second bag may be attached to receive used instruments which are
not of the disposable variety, or these may be placed in a special
receptacle.

A dressing pack may contain all equipment required, e.g. gauze
swabs, cotton wool mops, drapes, gallipots and forceps, or, alternatively, instruments and gallipots may be in their individual
packs.

Some additional requirements

Special individually wrapped dressings.

Disposable suture removal pack.

Sterile safety pins for securing drainage tubes.

Methylated ether for removal of adhesive strapping marks.

Sterile wound probe and sinus forceps.

Sterile packing material.

Antibiotic powder.

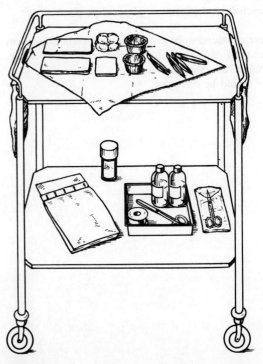

Figure 26
Trolley with basic requirements for surgical dressings

Clinical notes

Environmental hygiene:

Activities such as sweeping, dusting or bed-making should have ceased $\frac{1}{2}$ to 1 hour before the dressings are commenced.

The minimum of activity in the ward during dressings. Care with movement of bed curtains or screens, and bed clothes folded down with care, to minimise any increase in contamination of the air around the patient.

Understanding of the principles of the 'non-touch' technique and the importance of a carefully planned distribution of work within the 'dressing team'.

Order of procedure — 'clean' dressings first, then 'septic' ones.

Knowledge of dangers, methods, and prevention of 'cross infection' during wound dressing.

Importance of psychological as well as physical preparation of patients.

Minimum exposure of wound to be dressed, and of sterile equipment on the upper shelf of trolley after preparation at the bedside.

Care with disposal of all soiled materials.

Unused dressings should be discarded.

Notes

Intravenous (IV) infusion

This treatment may be necessary for a number of reasons which include the following:

To replace fluid loss and correct dehydration.

To maintain or correct serum electrolyte levels.

To maintain nutrition when the patient cannot be fed by other routes.

To maintain blood pressure and improve capillary circulation.

To provide the facility for administration of drugs into the venous system.

Requirements

A trolley cleaned and disinfected as for all sterile procedures.

The basic requirements as for surgical dressings plus:

Disposable giving set (including a filter if blood is to be given in the course of treatment).

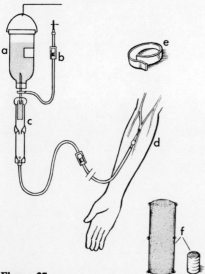

Figure 27

Intravenous infusion a. IV solution b. integral airway c. filter and drip chamber d. needle/cannula in antecubital vein e. arm band to facilitate distension of the vein f. padded arm splint and bandage

The needle, cannula or intracath.

Bottle or plastic container with the infusion fluid (this will depend on
the condition requiring treatment).

Sphygmomanometer.

Drip stand and bottle holder.

Sterile bowl to collect fluid which is run through giving set as it is
prepared for attachment to the IV needle.

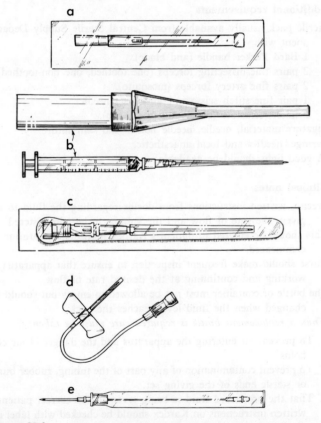

Figure 28.1
Intravenous cannulae   a. disposable IV needle   b. IV cannula (needle inside)
and syringe attached   c. IV cannula (Teflon) needle inside   d. 'Butterfly' intermittent infusion set with injection site   e. intracath (IV catheter inside
needle)

A suitable splint and bandage for the limb into which infusion is given.

Micropore tape.

Waterproof protection for bed.

A bed cradle should be available if leg vein is chosen for infusion.

It may sometimes be necessary to 'cut down' and expose the vein in order to introduce the cannula.

Additional requirements

Sterile pack usually available from Central Sterile Supply Department with:

    1 Bard Parker handle (and blade).

    2 pairs fine dissecting forceps (one toothed, one non-toothed).

    2 pairs fine artery forceps (mosquito).

    1 pair fine stitch scissors, 1 aneurysm needle.

    2 hook retractors (one blunt, one sharp).

Ligature material, needle, needle holder and skin suture.

Syringe, needles and local anaesthetic.

(A good light should be available)

Clinical notes

Precise, written instructions from doctor regarding the fluid to be given, the rate of flow and the volume to be administered.

This should be entered in patient's Kardex immediately infusion is commenced.

Nurse should make frequent inspection to ensure that apparatus is working and continuing at the desired rate of flow.

The bottle or container must not be allowed to empty but should be changed when the fluid level reaches the neck.

When a replacement bottle is required care must be taken:

1. To prevent air entering the apparatus and the danger of air embolus.

2. To prevent contamination of any part of the tubing, rubber bung or sterile ends of the giving set.

3. That the prescribed fluid is being given to the correct patient, written instructions on Kardex should be checked with label on bottle and witnessed by a qualified nurse.

4. That rate of flow is regulated after bottle has been changed.

5. To check that the container and the fluid show no obvious faults or contamination.

All fluids given must be recorded accurately on the patient's fluid balance chart.

Observation of the area around the point of insertion of needle for any leakage of fluid, swelling or inflammation.

In the event of difficulties, e.g. the infusion stopping or fluid running into the tissues, doctor should be informed.

Temperature, pulse and respiration should be recorded four hourly and blood pressure noted as requested.

It is preferable that drugs be added to infusion fluids by a doctor or pharmacist and this is recorded on the label of the container. In certain circumstances a registered nurse may be required to do so but only on the written instructions of a doctor who undertakes full responsibility for the procedure.

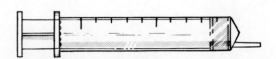

Figure 28.2
Disposable IV syringe (eccentric nozzle)

Subcutaneous infusion

This method may be chosen for the introduction of fluids in adults but is used more often in infants and young children. The infusion rate is slower than by the intravenous method and must be carefully controlled to ensure that it does not exceed the rate of absorption. Saline is the solution most commonly used as Dextrose is liable to cause irritation of the tissues and could lead to necrosis.

Requirements

The same basic equipment as for intravenous infusion and similar precautions to maintain sterility throughout procedure.

Add the following equipment

2 subcutaneous needles of suitable size.

Sterile Y connection, and two lengths of tubing, when two injection sites are to be used simultaneously.

Adaptors as required.

Ampoules of hyaluronidase (Hyalase), this is an enzyme which will help promote absorption of the fluid.

Syringe, needle and sterile distilled water.

Local anaesthetic, syringe and needles (when necessary).

A bed cradle should be available if required.

Note

Observation of the area is important for any leakage of fluid, hard swellings or blanching of the skin.

Sites chosen for the infusion may be on the outer aspect of the thigh, the abdominal wall and the axillary area.

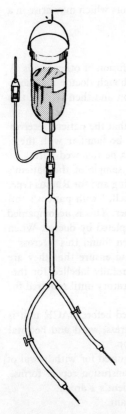

Figure 29
Apparatus for subcutaneous infusion

Blood transfusion

The circumstances in which this treatment will be necessary are numerous but the *indications for it fall into three main categories*.

The need to replace blood following haemorrhage and thus restore blood volume and blood pressure.

To increase the oxygen carrying facility as this is sometimes considerably reduced in anaemia.

The need for blood platelets and clotting factors which may arise in a disease such as haemophilia.

Requirements

These are similar to those for intravenous infusion of other fluids. A giving set with a filter must be used, though doctor may commence the infusion with a saline solution and then replace this with a unit of blood.

Special precautions must be taken to ensure that the patient receives blood of the correct group. Staff must be familiar with the routine procedure, which should always be followed with meticulous attention to every detail. A sample of the patient's blood is sent to the laboratory for grouping and for Rhesus type. This must be clearly and accurately labelled with patient's full name, address, ward and hospital number. This is accompanied by a request form which has been completed by doctor. When blood of the appropriate group has been found this is cross matched with the patient's own blood to ensure that they are compatible. The bottles or bags are carefully labelled for the specific patient and retained in the laboratory until required for use.

ALL IDENTIFYING DATA must be checked before EACH unit is transfused, i.e. patient's full name, address, ward and hospital number, bottle number and blood group.

Follow hospital procedure for signatures required for withdrawal of blood from bank and completion of transfusion report forms.

A precise record is always made in the patient's Kardex.

Close supervision of patient is most important.

Be on the alert for any incompatibility reaction, e.g. rigor, nausea, vomiting and pain in the lumbar region, and in such circumstances discontinue transfusion and inform doctor immediately.

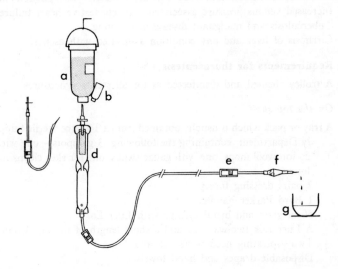

COMPATIBLE WITH
Patient's Name _____
Hospital _____ Ward _____ No _____
Blood Group _____ Date _____
Bottle No & Group _____
Place in Refrigerator until required

Figure 30
Blood transfusion a. bottle or pack with blood (see label) b. pilot bottle c. airway d. filter in drip set e. clamp f. injection site g. sterile bowl to collect fluid as air is expelled from apparatus h. padded arm splint (A similar administration set may be used for other fluids.)

Aspiration of the pleural cavity (thoracentesis)

Fluid may collect in the inter-pleural space in a number of conditions which include:

Irritation and inflammation of the pleura associated with pneumonia.

Increased venous pressure associated with congestive heart failure.

Tuberculosis and malignant disease of the lung.

Cirrhosis of liver and any condition associated with ascites.

Requirements for thoracentesis

A trolley cleaned and disinfected as for all sterile procedures.

On the top shelf

A tray or pack which is usually obtained from a Theatre Sterile Supply Department, containing the following: 3 gallipots – one with cotton wool mops, one with gauze swabs, one for skin cleansing lotion.

2 pairs dressing forceps.

1 Bard Parker handle.

50 ml glass and metal syringe with Luer Lok.

A Luer Lok two-way tap and a short length of tubing (15 cm).

Two aspirating needles size 16 and 17.

Disposable drapes and hand towels.

On the lower shelf

Face masks.

Sterile gown and gloves to be worn by doctor.

2 ml or 5 ml syringe and hypodermic needles size 23G and 21G.

Local anaesthetic, e.g. lignocaine (plain).

Skin disinfectant, e.g. Hibitane solution.

Blade for Bard Parker handle.

Sterile bowl.

Graduated jug, 1000 ml capacity.

Protection for bed.

Specimen bottle(s) as required.   Micropore tape.

Nobecutane spray.   (Two disposal bags attached to trolley).

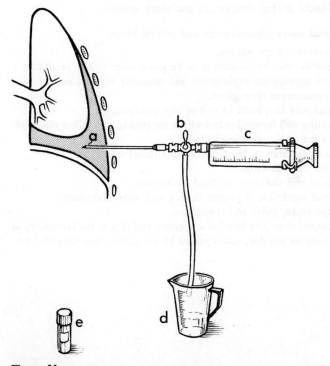

Figure 31
Aspiration of the pleural cavity (thoracentesis) a. aspirating needle b.
two way tap (Luer Lok) c. aspirating syringe d. graduated measure
e. laboratory specimen jar

Pleural biopsy

This may be undertaken to determine whether a pleural effusion is of malignant or tuberculous origin. It involves obtaining a small piece of the parietal pleura by using a special biopsy needle.

Requirements

Similar to those for thoracentesis with the addition of:
Abram's pleural biopsy needle.
Biopsy bottle.
Needle holder, skin suture and stitch scissors.

Clinical notes (thoracentesis and pleural biopsy)

Preparation of the patient:
A sedative may be prescribed to be given prior to the procedure.
Ensure appropriate explanation and adequate support and reassurance throughout.
Patient may be placed in one of two positions:
1. Sitting well forward in bed with arms resting on a pillow placed on a bed table, and head flexed.
2. Semi-recumbent, lying on the unaffected side.
Record the following:
Amount and character of fluid withdrawn.
General condition of patient during and after procedure.
Temperature, pulse and respiration.
Specimens should be labelled accurately and sent to the laboratory as soon as possible, accompanied by the appropriate request form.

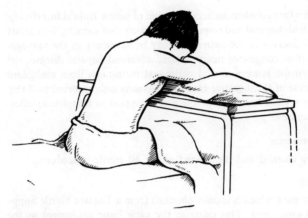

Figure 32.1
Position which may be used for pleural biopsy

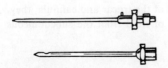

Figure 32.2
Abram's pleural biopsy needle

Abdominal paracentesis

This is performed when an accumulation of ascitic fluid is interfering with abdominal and respiratory function thus causing discomfort and distress to the patient. It may be necessary in the management of congestive heart failure, advanced hepatic disease, the nephrotic syndrome, and peritoneal metastases from malignant disease of the digestive tract. It is usually only resorted to if the ascitic fluid has failed to lessen or disappear in response to other measures.

Requirements

A trolley cleaned and disinfected as for all sterile procedures.

Top shelf

A tray or pack which is usually obtained from a Theatre Sterile Supply Department. This contains the same basic equipment as the thoracentesis pack but instead of aspiration needles and syringes:

A Metcalf or Thomson's ascites trocar and cannula.

A length of tubing to attach to cannula and long enough to reach the receptacle into which fluid is drained.

Lower shelf

Similar equipment as for thoracentesis plus:

A graduated drainage bag for fluid.

An abdominal binder.

Tape measure.

Gate clip.

Large safety pin to secure tubing to draw sheet.

Sphygmomanometer.

Two disposal bags attached to trolley.

(A stimulant tray should be available in case of collapse).

Southey's tubes may be used instead of the trocar and cannula, they may also be used for drainage of fluid from the subcutaneous tissues of the legs.

Clinical notes

Simple but adequate explanation to patient should include any instruction necessary and reassurance.

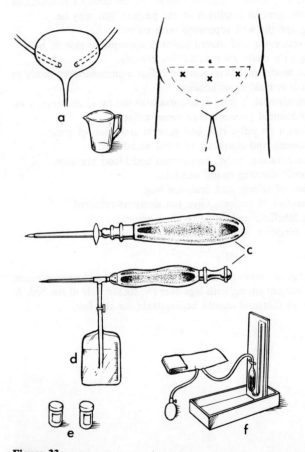

Figure 33

Abdominal paracentesis a. empty bladder b. possible sites for puncture c. types of trocar and cannula (Metcalf and Thomson's) d. graduated drainage bag e. laboratory specimen jars f. sphygmomanometer

The umbilicus, lower abdomen and groins must be thoroughly clean.

The area between the symphysis pubis and umbilicus is shaved when necessary.

Patient should empty bladder immediately before procedure.

Catheterisation may be needed as puncture of a distended bladder is the main danger to be avoided.

Positioning of patient – this will depend on the doctor's instructions and the general condition of the patient, but may be:

1. Sitting upright well supported with pillows.
2. Semi-recumbent and moved towards appropriate side of bed.
3. Sitting on a chair when condition permits.

Abdominal binder placed in position before commencement ready to tighten as fluid is withdrawn.

Rate of withdrawal of fluid is important as too rapid decrease of intra-abdominal pressure may cause collapse.

Careful watch on pulse rate and general condition of patient.

Record amount and character of fluid withdrawn.

Record temperature, pulse, respiration and blood pressure.

Secure sterile dressing round cannula.

Fix position of tubing and drainage bag.

Ensure comfort of patient. Give hot drink as required.

Attend to labelling and despatch of specimens.

Re-adjust binder as drainage continues.

Additional

For drainage of limbs ensure comfort and warmth and when possible have patient sitting with legs over the foot or side of the bed. A chair or footstool should be available for the feet.

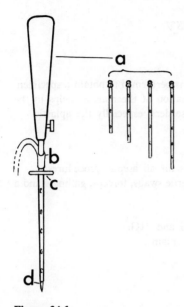

Figure 34.1
Southey's tubes a. tubes stored in handle when not in use b. trocar piercing tubing c. guard d. point of trocar

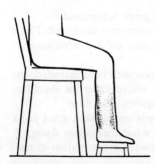

Figure 34.2
Position which may be used for drainage of fluid from lower limbs

Bone marrow biopsy

This is a diagnostic procedure and is performed to obtain a specimen of red bone marrow. Examination of the marrow helps in the diagnosis of certain blood disorders, especially the aplastic anaemias.

Requirements

Trolley cleaned and disinfected as for all aseptic procedures.

Large dressing pack containing sterile swabs, forceps, gallipots and a clinical sheet.

Packet with sterile drapes.

2 ml syringe and needles size 23G and 21G.

Local anaesthetic, e.g. lignocaine (plain).

Bottle with skin antiseptic.

10 ml aspirating syringe.

Nobecutane spray.

Micropore tape.

Haematology departments usually supply bone marrow needle, specimen containers or slides and fixative solution.

2 disposal bags attached to trolley.

Face mask and gown should be worn by doctor.

Clinical notes

Simple but adequate explanation given to patient as the procedure is not a pleasant one.

Doctor usually orders a sedative to be given beforehand.

The area may require to be shaved if the sternum is to be used. This is the commonest site in adults, although the iliac crest may sometimes be chosen.

Patient is placed in the recumbent position with head extended, one firm pillow only is used and this is placed under the shoulders.

Provide support and reassurance throughout procedure.

When puncture is sealed and patient made comfortable, a hot drink may be welcome as the treatment sometimes causes distress. Report on general condition and continue observation of the patient.

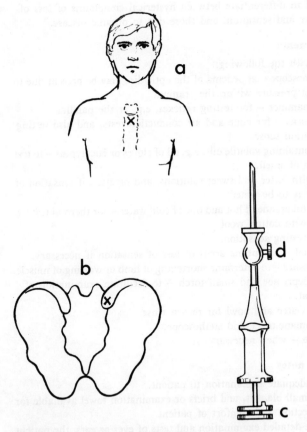

Figure 35
Bone marrow biopsy   a. sternal puncture site (opposite second intercostal space)   b. posterior superior iliac spine site   c. bone marrow biopsy needle
d. guard on needle

Neurological examination

Indications

Suspected disease or injury of the central nervous system. The need to investigate sensory perception, and motor and reflex activity.

The need to differentiate between hysterical complaints of loss of power and sensation, and those due to organic disease.

Requirements

Trolley with the following:

Ophthalmoscope – as oedema of the optic disc may be present due to rising pressure within the cranium.

Tendon hammer – for testing reflexes, e.g. at the patella.

Tuning forks – for bone and air conduction tests, and also testing vibration sense.

Bottles containing volatile oils, e.g. oil of cloves or eucalyptus – to test sense of smell.

Bottles with bitter and sweet solutions, and pipettes, if sensation of taste is to be tested.

Two test tubes, one of hot and one of cold water – for thermal testing.

Gallipot with cotton wool.

Pins for testing sensation.

Skin pencil – to outline areas of loss of sensation if necessary.

Tape measure – to determine shortening of limb or wasting of muscle.

Tongue depressor and small torch – to facilitate examination of throat.

Glass of water and bowl for return rinse.

Sphygmomanometer and stethoscope.

Auriscope – when necessary.

Clinical notes

Ensure adequate explanation to patient.

Have a small blanket, and briefs or examination towel available for protection and comfort of patient.

For some detailed examination and tests of eyes or ears, the patient may be taken to the appropriate department.

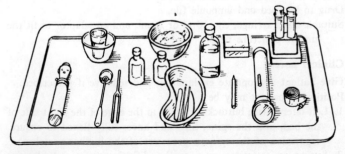

Figure 36
Tray for neurological examination

Lumbar puncture

Indications

To obtain specimens of cerebro-spinal fluid (CSF) for examination and analysis.

To measure pressure of CSF and sometimes to withdraw some CSF to relieve intra-cranial pressure.

To introduce drugs intrathecally for therapeutic or diagnostic purposes.

Requirements

Trolley cleaned and disinfected as for all aseptic procedures.

A tray or pack is usually available from a Central Sterile Supply Department containing 2 lumbar puncture needles, spinal manometer, two-way tap (if not already incorporated in needles), length of tubing to connect manometer to two-way tap.

Dressings pack containing swabs, gallipots, forceps and clinical sheet.

Packet of sterile drapes.

2 ml syringe and 2 needles size 23G and 21G.

Local anaesthetic, e.g. lignocaine (plain).

Skin antiseptic, Nobecutane spray, micropore tape.

Specimen bottles as required – usually 3.

Face masks and also packet with sterile gloves when necessary.

Two disposal bags attached to trolley.

When a drug is to be injected, e.g. an antibiotic, or a radio-opaque substance such as Myodil, add:

Drug to be used and ampoule file.

Suitable sized syringe, e.g. 10 ml or 20 ml, and an adaptor to fit the lumbar puncture needle.

Clinical notes

Give patient appropriate explanation and sedative if prescribed.

Position of patient may be:

1. Left lateral with buttocks brought to the edge of the right side of the bed, and the spine, hips and knees fully flexed to ensure separation of the spinous processes of the lumbar vertebrae.

2. Sitting up (sometimes on a stool) and flexing the spine by leaning forward with head towards knees and well supported by nurse.

Two people should help support the patient and avoid any sudden movement as needle is inserted (usually between third and fourth lumbar vertebrae). *Queckenstedt's test* may be performed when the pressure of the CSF is being recorded. This is done by applying pressure to the jugular vein and noting any rise in CSF pressure.

Always observe general condition of patient throughout procedure and report any complaint of pain, headache or nausea.

Attend to labelling of specimens and despatch to laboratory in an upright position.

Patient should rest with head low for six to twelve hours after procedure. It may be helpful to elevate the foot of the bed to prevent headache.

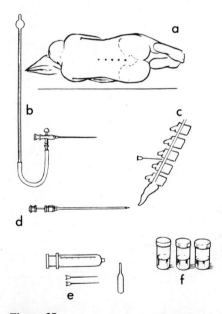

Figure 37
Lumbar puncture   a. position which may be used for lumbar puncture   b. spinal manometer, tubing, two-way tap and spinal needle   c. site of puncture, between third and fourth lumbar vertebrae   d. spinal needle with stilette withdrawn   e. requisites for introducing local anaesthetic   f. laboratory specimen jars

Cisternal puncture

The CSF may also be tapped at the space known as the cisterna magna. The needle used is shorter than a lumbar puncture needle and is graduated in centimetres to enable accurate control of the depth of penetration. It is introduced between the first cervical vertebra (the atlas) and the base of the skull (the occiput). The equipment used is otherwise similar to that for lumbar puncture. The site should be shaved at the back of the neck and up to the occipital protruberance. The patient is usually sitting up with neck well flexed and head supported, but the lateral position may be adopted when necessary.

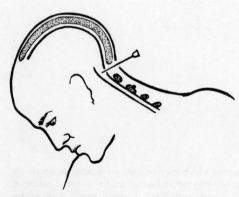

Figure 38
Site for cisternal puncture

Electroplexy

Modified electro-convulsive therapy (ECT) has become an integral part of treatment in psychiatric hospitals. It is an effective adjunct to appropriate drug treatment of severe depression.

Indications for ECT

Severe suicidal tendencies.

Melancholic states.

Post-menopausal depression in women and climacteric depression in men.

Manic depressive reaction.

Acute psychotic episodes in schizophrenia.

Two trolleys are usually prepared with the equipment.

One for the anaesthetist and one for the actual ECT.

Trolley for anaesthetist

The drugs to be administered.

Sterile syringes and needles:

2 ml syringe for atropine sulphate.

10 ml syringe for thiopentone sodium (Pentothal).

5 ml syringe for suxamethonium chloride (Anectine)

Intravenous needles 23G x 3.5 cm.

A 'mixing' needle when necessary and an ampoule of sterile water for injection.

Swabs impregnated with a skin disinfectant (Mediswab) or cotton wool mops and a gallipot containing, for example, skin Hibitane.

An artificial airway ('Portex' disposable).

Mouth gag.

Clinical sheet or drape.

Disposal bag.

In addition:

> Tourniquet.
> Oxygen cylinder and tubing.
> Ambu bag.
> Suction apparatus.

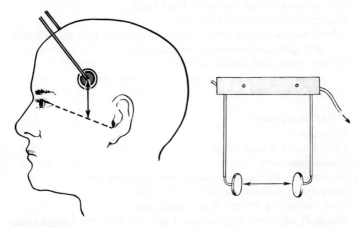

Figure 39.1
Electroplexy – bilateral method. Head band in use and electrode in position
5 cm above the mid-point of a line drawn from the lateral angle of the eye to
external auditory meatus

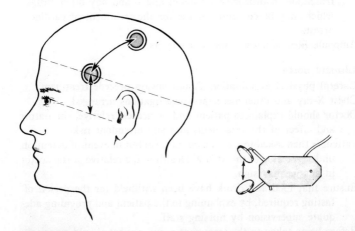

Figure 39.2
Electroplexy – unilateral method. Head band in use and electrodes placed,
one on the temporal region 4 cm above the mid-point of the eye/ear line and
the other above the ear 6 cm from the first and over the parietal region

105

Trolley for ECT

The electroplexy machine with head band.

Electrodes covered with white lint.

A bowl with electrolyte solution in which electrode pads are well soaked before commencement of treatment.

Oxygen masks and anaesthetic face masks.

Tongue depressor, tongue forceps and mouth 'bite'.

Receptacle for used items.

Other equipment

Laryngoscope.

Cuffed endotracheal tubes.

Suction catheters.

Stethoscope, sphygmomanometer and diagnostic set.

Intravenous infusion set and IV cannulae.

Pack containing IV 'cut down' equipment.

Sterile IV solutions, e.g. dextrose 5 per cent W/V and sodium bicarbonate 8.4 per cent W/V.

Assorted sterile disposable syringes and needles.

A sealed tray with emergency drugs:

Adrenaline; atropine sulphate; aminophylline; nikethamide; frusemide; hydrocortisone; lignocaine – and any other drugs which may be currently in use for the treatment of cardiac arrest.

Ampoule files, adhesive tape and scissors.

Clinical notes

Careful physical examination should always precede treatment.

Chest X-ray and other necessary investigations arranged.

Doctor should explain to patient and/or nearest relative, the nature and effect of the treatment, and any attendant risks.

Patient is then asked to sign a consent form but in event of detention under a section of the Mental Health Act, a relative or the doctor in charge may sign.

Ensure that food and drink have been withheld for the period of fasting required, by explaining to the patient and providing adequate supervision by nursing staff.

Before being taken to the treatment room, patient should empty the bladder (and bowel if necessary).

Tight clothing round neck, chest and waist is loosened, shoes must be removed.

Hair grips and all cosmetics are removed.

Dentures, spectacles and jewellery should be labelled and placed in 'safe keeping' according to hospital rules.

Following the treatment

Patient's lungs are ventilated with oxygen until spontaneous breathing is re-established and this usually occurs in three to five minutes. Patient is placed in the semi-prone position.

On regaining consciousness the patient may be restless, confused or emotional and is kept under close observation. Any signs of cyanosis or respiratory distress should be reported immediately.

The pulse is checked and recorded as instructed.

When fully recovered, the patient should be provided with toilet facilities. Items which were placed in 'safe keeping' are returned.

A cup of tea and the necessary support and reassurance should be given.

If the patient is an out-patient, the hospital rules regarding fitness for discharge and any arrangements for transport should be adhered to at all times.

Peritoneal dialysis

Indications for treatment

Acute or chronic renal failure, when the aim is to replace or complement the work of the kidneys when they are unable to function adequately.

Acute poisoning, to facilitate extraction of the poison, e.g. salicylates or some of the shorter acting barbiturates.

Some cases of severe heart failure, when this may be considered a suitable method of removing water from the patient.

Requirements

Trolley cleaned and disinfected as for all aseptic procedures.

Dressings pack containing swabs, gallipot, forceps and drapes.

Packet with sterile Bard Parker handle, trocar and cannula.

Scalpel blade.

Abdominal catheter set, i.e. a many-eyed, semi-rigid nylon catheter and guide.

Local anaesthetic, e.g. lignocaine (plain).

Syringes, 2 ml and 5 ml, and needles, 23G and 21G.

Peritoneal administration set.

Two 1 litre plastic packs with dialysing solution – these are warmed to body temperature.

Skin antiseptic.

Receptacle(s) for return of fluid from the peritoneal cavity.

Ampoules of potassium chloride (this is added to the dialysate according to needs of the patient).

Heparin. A small amount may be added to dialysate to decrease chance of clot formation in catheter.

Two disposal bags attached to trolley.

Sterile gown, mask and gloves for doctor.

Infusion stand at bedside.

Clinical notes

Adequate explanation to, and preparation of, the patient.

Consent form signed by patient or relative.

A mild sedative may be necessary to allay anxiety.

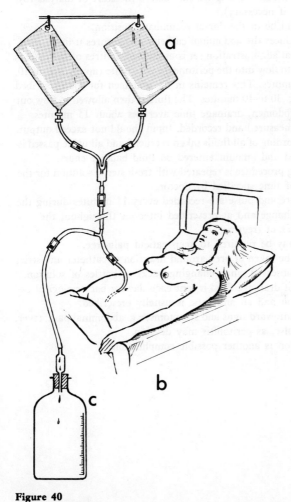

Figure 40
Peritoneal dialysis
a. two 1 litre packs of dialysate b. note position of catheter in peritoneal cavity c. a 2 litre collecting bottle

Prior to treatment, doctor will ascertain blood levels of electrolytes, urea and creatinine.

Weight, blood pressure and pulse are recorded.

The bladder should be emptied just before the start of dialysis (by catheter if necessary).

Patient should be in the dorsal recumbant position.

Doctor introduces the abdominal catheter and secures it in position.

The peritoneal administration set is assembled. 2 litres of dialysate is allowed to flow into the peritoneal cavity quite rapidly, e.g. in 10 to 15 minutes. This remains in the abdomen for the prescribed time, e.g. 30 to 40 minutes. The fluid is then allowed to flow out of the abdomen, drainage time averages about 15 minutes.

Drainage is measured and recorded. Input should not exceed output.

Accurate recording of all fluids taken is crucial and all urine passed is measured and amount entered on fluid balance chart.

The dialysing procedure is repeated with fresh sterile solution for the period of time specified by doctor.

Blood pressure and pulse are recorded every 15 minutes during the first exchange and at prescribed intervals throughout the remainder of treatment.

Analgesics may be required to keep patient pain-free.

Care should be taken of area around insertion of catheter and strict asepsis observed when changing packs or bottles of solution.

A specimen of drainage fluid is sent each day for bacteriological examination and an antibiotic is usually prescribed.

Report any untoward signs and symptoms, e.g. abdominal pain, fever, rapid pulse, as peritonitis may develop.

Chest infection is another possible complication.

Underwater seal drainage

In thoracic surgery when the pleural cavity has been opened, the surgeon may leave one or two inter-costal tubes in the pleural space when he closes the chest wall. This allows drainage of fluid, blood and air, and facilitates re-expansion of lung. The distal end of the drainage tube(s) is connected to the long glass tube which passes through the stopper of the drainage bottle and underneath the surface of the water, thus preventing air entering the thoracic cavity. If air is allowed to enter the pleural space, this causes atelectasis and endangers life. The short tube which passes through the stopper acts as an air outlet. The bottle should contain a measured amount of sterile water thus enabling the amount of drainage to be calculated. Drainage is assisted by the patient's own respiratory movements and provided the inter-costal tube remains patent, the water level in the glass tube will be seen to oscillate, rising with inspiration and falling again with expiration. A system which uses two bottles and a means of suction may also be used to facilitate drainage.

The underwater seal drainage may also be used in some cases of spontaneous pneumothorax although a *Heimlich valve* may be preferred. This is a 'one way' valve and is attached to a plastic drainage bag. It has the advantage that the patient can be allowed a considerable degree of mobility.

Clinical notes

Nurse must understand the reasons for the use of 'water-seal' drainage and also the principles on which the system operates. Bottle(s) must be situated below the level of the patient's chest. They are usually placed in a 'safe area' on the floor.

A bottle must never be lifted to chest level without first making sure that the tubing is clamped, otherwise fluid from the bottle will be siphoned into the pleural space.

Two pairs of tubing clamps should be kept at the bedside and be applied before any adjustments such as removal of stopper(s) and emptying or changing bottle(s). They must also be applied immediately in case of any emergency such as a bottle being accidentally knocked over (every effort should be made to avoid

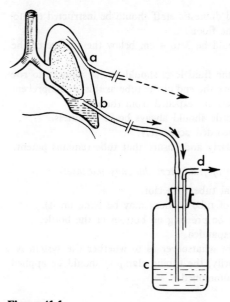

Figure 41.1
One bottle system of underwater seal drainage
a. apical tube to underwater seal allows escape of air   b. basal tube to underwater seal allows escape of sero-sanguinous fluid   c. water seal   d. air vent

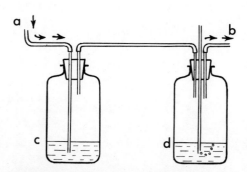

Figure 41.2
Two bottle system of water seal drainage with use of suction   a. from intercostal tube.   b. to suction.   c. drainage and sterile water   d. sterile water

such a situation and domestic staff should be instructed not to lift a bottle from the floor).

The long glass tube should be 3 to 4 cm below the surface of the water.

As drainage continues, the fluid level should not be allowed to rise more than 6 cm above the end of the tube as this would prevent air from being effectively expelled from the chest.

A sterile replacement bottle should always be in readiness.

All drainage must be recorded accurately.

Check connections regularly and ensure that tube remains patent.

If there is no oscillation of fluid level this may indicate:

1. Blocking of intercostal tube with clot.
2. Twisting or kinking of tube (patient may be lying on it).
3. Long glass tube may be pressing on bottom of the bottle.
4. Lung may be fully expanded.

When there is any doubt whatsoever as to whether the system is operating satisfactorily, the tubing clamp(s) should be applied and medical help summoned.

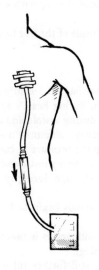

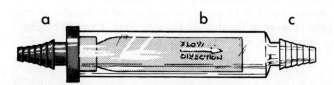

Figure 41.3
Heimlich valve a. attached to intra-pleural catheter b. one-way valve c. attached to tubing leading to drainage bag

Measurement of arterial blood pressure

The arterial blood pressure is measured in man by means of a *sphygmomanometer*.

This consists of a rubber bag (covered with a cloth envelope) which is wrapped round the upper arm over the brachial artery.

One tube connects the inside of the bag with a manometer containing mercury.

Another tube connects the inside of the bag to a hand-operated pump with a release valve.

Method

Air is pumped into the rubber bag till pressure in cuff is greater than pressure in artery even during heart's systole.

Artery is then closed down during systole and diastole. At same time air is pushing up mercury column in manometer.

By releasing valve on pump the pressure in cuff is gradually reduced till maximum pressure in artery just overcomes pressure in cuff.

Some blood begins to spurt through during systole, artery still closed during diastole.

Faint rhythmical tapping sounds begin to be heard through stethoscope.

The height of mercury in millimetres is taken as the *systolic blood pressure* (e.g. 120 mmHg).

Pressure in cuff is reduced still further till it is just less than the lowest pressure in artery towards the end of diastole (i.e. just before next heart beat).

Blood flow is unimpeded during systole and diastole.

The sounds stop. The height of mercury in the manometer at this point is taken as the *diastolic blood pressure* (about 80 mmHg).

These values differ with sex, age, exercise, sleep, etc.

(Taken from McNaught & Callander, 1975, *Illustrated Physiology*, p.93. Edinburgh: Churchill Livingstone)

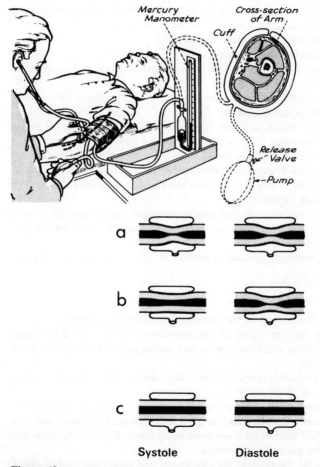

Figure 42
Measurement of arterial blood pressure (McNaught and Callander, 1975) a. artery closed during systole and diastole b. blood spurts through during systole, artery closed during diastole c. unimpeded blood flow.

117

Central venous pressure

The measurement of central venous pressure (CVP) enables the physician to estimate how the circulating blood volume compares to the pumping action of the heart at any given time.

Monitoring of CVP may be indicated:

1. Following cardiac surgery.
2. When estimating a safe volume of fluid replacement following surgery or severe injuries.
3. To enable differentiation between congestive heart failure and hypovolaemic shock.

A trolley which has been cleaned and disinfected as for all aseptic procedures is set with the following sterile equipment.

Basic requirements as for intravenous infusion.

The special intravenous catheter to be used (this is introduced via the basilic or jugular vein into the superior vena cava and into the right atrium).

A three way stopcock (for attachment to the tubing from the infusion set and that from the catheter, and also to the manometer).

A water manometer.

The prescribed solution to be used in order to keep the vein open.

Clinical notes

When a CVP reading is to be taken:

Have the patient in the recumbent position if possible.

Adjust the zero point on the manometer to the level of the right atrium which may be marked on the patient's skin by the physician.

The stopcock is opened to allow the manometer to fill with fluid to a level of 30 to 35 cm.

The stopcock is adjusted again to close off the flow from the intravenous bottle and permit a flow between manometer and vein.

The fluid level in the manometer being noted. It should fluctuate with the patient's respiration.

When the fluctuations are rhythmical and steady the reading should be taken. The highest level of the fluid column is recorded.

The stopcock is again adjusted to allow the infusion of the intravenous solution to continue.

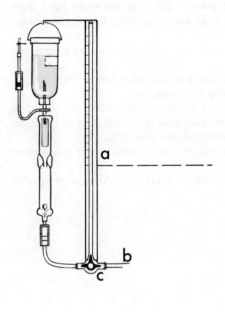

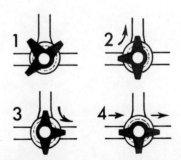

Figure 43
Measurement of central venous pressure a. zero on manometer tube on level with right atrium b. tubing to vein c. stopcock
Stopcock positions 1. closed 2. open to manometer tube 3. flow from manometer to vein 4. from solution bottle to vein

Frequency of recordings will depend on physician's instructions.

The normal range of CVP is approximately 5 to 10 cm of water. *A high or rising CVP*, e.g. 15 to 20 cm, indicates predominant cardiac failure when the blood is being returned to the right heart more rapidly than the heart can pump it into the arterial circulation.

Pulmonary oedema may occur, and rate and volume of intravenous fluids is adjusted.

A low or falling CVP indicates a serious reduction in blood volume and fluid repletion may be necessary.

If there has been a significant change in the reading, the physician should be informed. He may have given indication of the levels which will call for his immediate attention.

Measurement of arterial blood pressure is carried out in conjunction with CVP readings.

Observation and care of the site of insertion of the catheter must be maintained.

Notes

Catheterisation of the urinary bladder

This may be necessary for any of the following reasons:

Pre-operatively to ensure an empty bladder.

Post-operatively to prevent contamination of the operation area and avoid urinary complications.

For relief of retention of urine.

To facilitate bladder wash-out, and drainage and removal of blood clot following operation, e.g. prostatectomy.

Withdrawal and measurement of residual urine.

To obtain an uncontaminated specimen of urine for bacteriological examination (when it is not possible to procure a mid-stream specimen).

To facilitate diagnosis and treatment when patient is comatose.

Requirements

Trolley cleaned and disinfected as for all aseptic procedures.

A large dressing pack with the following sterile materials, cotton wool mops, gauze swabs, gallipot, two pairs forceps, drapes and clinical sheet.

Packet with sterile receptacle for collecting urine.

Sterile lubricant, e.g. liquid paraffin or catheter jelly.

Antiseptic lotion for swabbing, e.g. Hibitane 0.1 per cent.

Bowl for swabbing lotion.

Two pre-packed sterile catheters, e.g. of disposable nelaton type.

Specimen container.

Graduated jug for measuring urine.

Anglepoise lamp.

Sterile gloves (when preferred).

Sterile scissors to cut catheter packs.

Two disposal bags attached to the trolley.

Face masks, caps and gowns to be worn by nurses.

Add the following if a self retaining catheter is to be used:

Foley catheter (or alternative choice).

Sterile water to inflate balloon and a 5 ml or 10 ml syringe.

Drainage bag as required.

Sterile spigot if necessary.

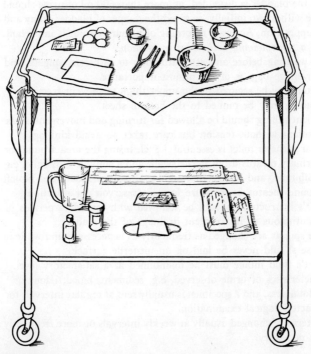

Figure 44.1
Trolley for catheterisation of the urinary bladder

For catheterisation of male patient: same basic requirements, suitable length and type of catheters should be available.

Addition of sterile urethral local anaesthetic may be necessary.

Clinical notes

It is essential to appreciate the dangers associated with this procedure. Precautions must be taken to avoid introducing micro-organisms into the urinary tract.

Preliminary cleansing of the genitalia must be thorough.

Strict aseptic technique for introduction of the catheter, which should be inserted into the urethra with sterile-gloved hands or using sterile forceps, taking care that it does not touch any external part.

Poor technique and the use of unsuitable catheters may cause trauma.

When the bladder is distended, no more than 600 ml of urine should be withdrawn initially, to avoid the danger of bladder atony and suppression. Accurate recording of urinary output is important.

When a self-retaining catheter is in position:

Hand washing before and after attention to catheters, spigots, and drainage bags is of the utmost importance.

Catheter may be secured to the upper thigh to prevent traction, or tubing may be pinned to the bottom sheet.

Sufficient tubing should be allowed for turning and movement of the patient without tension but care taken to avoid kinking.

Regular catheter toilet is essential, i.e. cleansing the area around the urinary meatus using sterile swabs and a suitable antiseptic, e.g. Hibitane, and drying thoroughly. Dressings should not be left round meatus as moisture forms a reservoir for infection.

Doctor's instructions should be followed with regard to periods of continuous or intermittent drainage of the bladder.

Sterile spigots are changed as frequently as is necessary and while in use should never be laid on an unsterile surface.

Patient's fluid intake must be maintained at a satisfactory level.

Characteristics of urine observed, e.g. sediment, blood, odour or cloudiness, and a specimen is usually sent at regular intervals for bacteriological examination.

Catheters are changed usually at weekly intervals or more frequently if necessary.

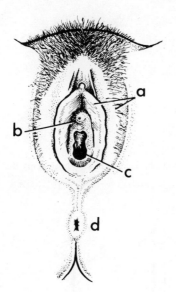

Figure 44.2
External genitalia a. labia
b. urethral meatus c. vaginal
orifice d. anus

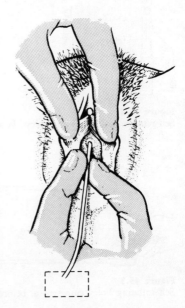

Figure 44.3
Female catheterisation. The catheter is inserted with sterile-gloved
hand (sterile forceps may be
used), the other end of the catheter
is in a sterile receptacle.

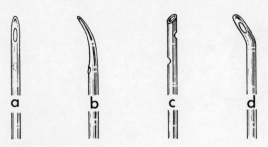

Figure 45.1
Urethral catheters a. Standard/Nelaton b. Tiemann c. Whistle Tip d. Coudé

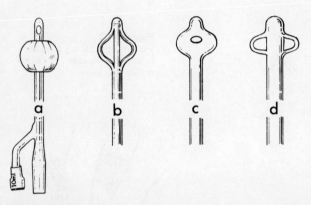

Figure 45.2
Self-retaining catheters a. Foley b. Dowse c. DePezzer d. Malecot

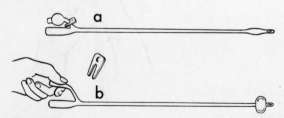

Figure 45.3
Self inflating Foley catheter a. before inflation b. inflating the balloon

Bladder drainage

This may be carried out by any one of the following methods:

1. Simple drainage by gravity

The self retaining catheter is attached by a sterile connection to the
tubing of a sterile, closed, urine collecting bag which is graduated
(Urisac). This is suspended from the bed frame using a metal or
plastic hanger. The tubing should be fixed to the lower sheet,
allowing for movement of the patient and also preventing kinking of the tube.

Drainage may be continuous or intermittent.

2. Closed drainage with additional facilities for irrigation

The self retaining catheter has a sterile Y connection inserted into the
lumen of the tube. One limb of the Y is attached to the tubing of
the sterile, closed, urine collecting bag and the second limb is
connected to a sterile drip set with a bottle or bag of the appropriate irrigating fluid attached. Gate clamps are attached to
both limb tubes.

When irrigation is desired

The clip on the tube leading to the drainage bag is closed.

The clip on the tube from the drip set is opened and 160 to 200 ml of
fluid is allowed to run into the bladder then the clip is again closed.

The clip on the drainage tube is opened thus allowing the irrigating
fluid and any debris to be washed out of the bladder.

When considerable irrigation is necessary, the urine collecting bag
may be replaced by a large sterile glass bottle suitable for a larger
volume of fluid.

It is sometimes necessary to gently irrigate the bladder using a
bladder syringe in order to dislodge clots which may be forming
post-operatively.

3. Combined supra-pubic and urethral drainage

This may be used in the immediate post-operative period to prevent
clot retention after operation on the bladder. It is discontinued

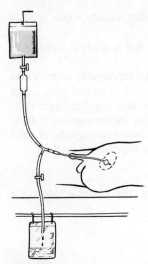

Figure 46
Closed drainage and bladder irrigation

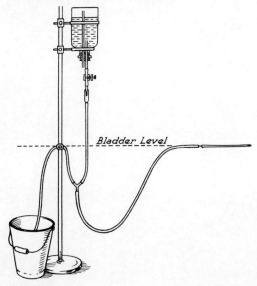

Bladder Level

Figure 47
Tidal drainage

when clot formation has been controlled, usually within 24 to 48 hours.

The patient has a supra-pubic catheter and a urethral catheter in position.

Lotion from a drip set passes through the supra-pubic catheter into the bladder and is drained out along with urine and other debris via the urethral catheter into the drainage bag. See figure 48.1.

The same principle may operate by altering the connections to allow fluid from the drip set to enter the bladder through the urethral catheter and be drained out via the supra-pubic catheter.

4. Tidal drainage

This may be used when necessary to help restore muscle tone to the bladder.

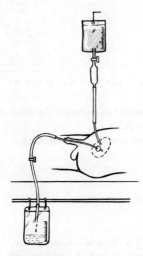

Figure 48.1
Combined supra-pubic and urethral bladder drainage

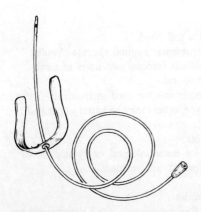

Figure 48.2
Gibbon catheter with retaining wings and adaptor

Vaginal examination

Indications for this procedure

Diagnosis of gynaecological conditions, e.g. tumours or displacements of the uterus.

To diagnose pregnancy and in the later months to ascertain the stage of labour and presenting part of the fetus.

To obtain specimens for bacteriological or cytological examination.

Requirements

Tray with the following:

Disposable gloves and a lubricant, e.g. obstetric cream.

Perineal pad and disposal bag.

Clinical sheet.

The above may be all that is necessary for a *bimanual examination*, i.e. two fingers of the right hand inserted into the vagina and palpation of the lower abdomen with the left hand.

When a more extensive and visual examination is to be carried out and especially during labour, following abortion or child birth, and after gynaecological surgery, *a trolley with sterile equipment* will be required.

Vaginal dressing pack containing cotton wool mops, gauze swabs, perineal pad and drapes.

Sterile gloves.

Jug with swabbing lotion and a foil bowl.

A tray with the necessary instruments: vaginal specula (Sim's, Cusco's, Ferguson's), volsellum forceps, two pairs of swab holding forceps, a uterine sound.

A disposal bag and suitable receptacle for used instruments (some specula are of disposable type, others may be battery operated to provide illumination).

A good light should be available.

When specimens are required for bacteriological or cytological examination additional equipment will include:

Cervical swab or long pipette.

Microscope slides or culture media.

Ayre's spatula, glass slide and fixative solution, for Papanicolaou examination ('Pap' Test). See figure 52.

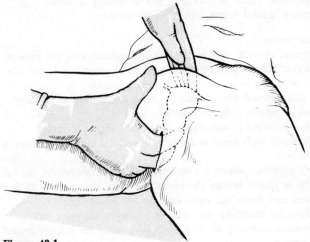

Figure 49.1
Bi-manual vaginal examination

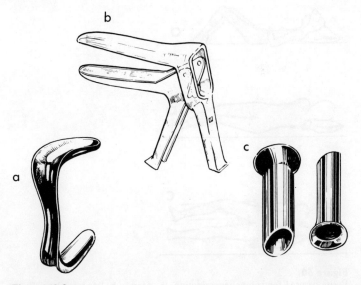

Figure 49.2
Types of vaginal specula in use a. Sim's b. Cusco's (disposable) c. Ferguson's

All specimens should be carefully and accurately labelled.
Laboratory request forms completed by doctor.

Clinical notes

Appropriate physical and psychological preparation of the patient.
Ensure that bladder is emptied just prior to examination. It may also
be necessary to ensure that rectum is empty.
Pubic and perineal area should be clean and shaved as required.
Position of patient (Fig.50) may be:

1. Dorsal recumbent with knees flexed and thighs abducted.
2. Left lateral with knees and thighs flexed and buttocks at edge of
the bed.
3. Sim's position – which is a modification of the left lateral, the left
arm is placed behind the patient and she lies forward on her
chest and flexes the right knee above the left one.

Procedure for swabbing the vulva is as for vulval toilet but *no
previous cleansing* when a swab is required for bacteriological
purposes.

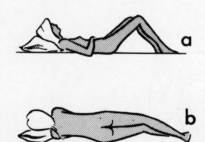

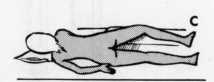

Figure 50
Positions used for vaginal examination   a. dorsal   b. left lateral   c. Sim's
position

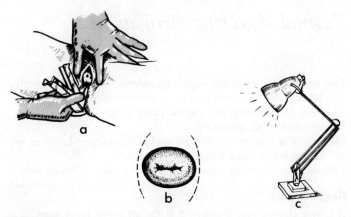

Figure 51
Visual examination of the vagina
a. Cusco's speculum being introduced into the vagina
b. cervix of uterus viewed through speculum
c. a good light available

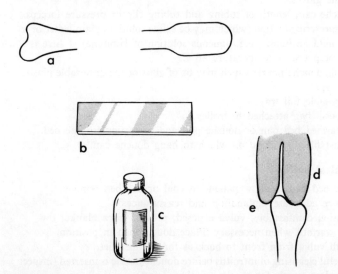

Figure 52
Specimen for cytological examination a. Ayre's spatula b. glass slide c. fixative solution d. uterus e. part of spatula rotated to procure specimen

Vaginal douching (irrigation)

This treatment is much less frequently ordered than it was formerly.
When it is considered necessary, the *indications for it include:*
The need for cleansing the vaginal canal before certain
gynaecological operations.
Presence of a profuse or offensive vaginal discharge which has not
responded to other forms of treatment.
The need for cleansing when a supportive pessary is being worn.

Requirements

A trolley cleaned and disinfected as for all sterile procedures.
Sterile vaginal dressing pack containing cotton wool mops, gauze
swabs, perineal pad and drape.
Jug with warmed swabbing lotion, e.g. Hibitane 1:2000.
Large sterile foil bowl.
Sterile gloves.
Douche can, length of tubing and tubing clip or pressure forceps.
The prescribed lotion (which may be saline solution, plain water or a
mild antiseptic, e.g. aqueous solution of Hibitane). 1 litre is
prepared at temperature 40°C.
Sterile douche nozzle which may be of glass or the disposable plastic
type.
Disposable foil tray.
Disposal bag attached to trolley.
A warmed bed pan or douche pan and protection for the bed.
Adjustable drip stand on which to hang douche can.

Clinical notes

Give bed pan to allow patient to void urine, then remove.
Ensure adequate explanation and reassurance.
Position comfortably, vulva exposed, provide extra blanket for
warmth when necessary. Place douche pan in position.
Swab vulva from front to back as for vulval toilet.
Careful cleansing of introitus before douche nozzle is inserted (inspect
glass nozzle for cracks or other defect).
Douche can should be suspended 25 to 30 cm above the pelvis to allow
gentle irrigation at low pressure.

Patient should sit up on douche pan and be encouraged to cough before pan is removed. Ensure that vulva, perineum and cleft of buttocks are thoroughly dried before applying fresh pad as required.

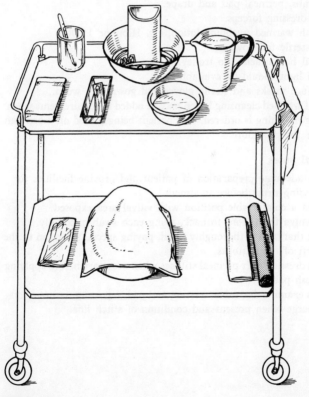

Figure 53
Trolley for vaginal douching

Vulval toilet and perineal care

This forms a routine part of obstetric nursing care following child birth and is also necessary after certain gynaecological operations.

Requirements

Trolley cleaned and disinfected as for all sterile procedures.
Sterile vaginal dressing pack containing cotton wool mops, gauze swabs, perineal pad and drape.
Sterile dressing forceps.
Jug with warmed swabbing lotion, e.g. Hibitane 1:2000.
Large sterile foil bowl.
Disposal bag attached to trolley.
A good light should be available.
Caps, face masks and sterile gloves and gowns are worn.
A jug of warmed cleansing lotion may be added to requirements when jug douching is ordered. The patient being placed on a bed pan for the procedure.

Clinical notes

Ensure adequate preparation of patient and provide facilities for voiding urine before treatment.
Place in a comfortable position with vulval area exposed.
Swab vulva from front to back, using each swab once only.
Ensure that area is thoroughly dried, paying special attention to the cleft of the buttocks.
Place a dressing over perineal stitches when necessary before applying fresh pad.
Always examine discarded dressing and pad, reporting nature of discharge when present and condition of stitch line.

Insertion of medicated pessaries

These may be prescribed in the treatment of a number of conditions affecting the vagina. They are soluble preparations which may contain antibiotics, antifungal agents, oestrogens or lactic acid.

Requirements

Tray with the following:
The prescribed pessary.
Disposable gloves.
Swabs for cleansing.
Disposal bag.
Vulval pad if necessary.

Clinical notes

Give adequate explanation to patient.
Ensure that opportunity is given to void urine.
Position comfortably in either the left lateral or dorsal position with knees drawn up.
Ensure that pessary is introduced as far as possible into the posterior fornix of the vagina.
Patient should remain in bed for one hour after insertion of pessary in the morning and the last one should be inserted after retiral to bed in the evening.
Nurse should always check prescription sheet.

Application of plaster of Paris

This material is used very frequently for external splintage of different parts of the body and it is applied for a variety of purposes.

To immobilise injured limbs as in fractures or severe sprains.

To prevent or correct deformity.

To provide rest for a part and permit healing to take place.

Requirements

A trolley with the following:

Tray with the requisite number and widths of plaster bandages.

Tray with stockinet of suitable width for limb or trunk, cotton wool bandages, any other felt or sorbo which may be necessary for padding, and a pair of dressing scissors.

Open wove cotton bandages.

A tin of dry plaster, jug of warm water and a bowl, when plaster cream is required, e.g. in preparation of some plaster shells to treat injury or disease of the spine.

Jar of glove powder.

A tape measure and skin pencil.

A lubricant for application to the skin in preparation for making, for instance, a plaster bed.

Plaster shears and knives (when an old plaster is to be removed, an electric saw may be used).

A bucket or large bowl with tepid water and deep enough to permit adequate soaking of plaster bandages.

Any appliance which is to be incorporated in the plaster, e.g. walking iron, heel, rocker or Cramer wire.

A board or other smooth working surface for preparation of slabs.

Protection for floor, and bed or treatment area.

Rubber gloves, waterproof aprons and rubber boots or canvas overboots for protection of surgeon and other plaster room staff.

Protect patient's clothing.

Fracture boards under mattress and large bed cradle available when necessary.

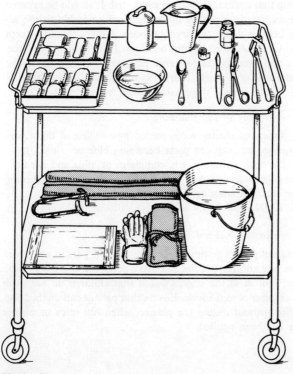

Figure 54
Trolley for application of plaster of Paris

Clinical notes

The plaster is usually applied by the surgeon, a trained technician or an experienced nurse. The art is only acquired by experience under well supervised and skilled tuition.

When the hand or arm is involved, rings or other jewellery are removed. During application the limb must be held steady and in the correct position (usually that of function unless otherwise indicated by the surgeon).

The completed plaster is usually dated and initialled by the person who applied it and the patient is given instructions on exercises and general care of plaster (these are in writing for the outpatient, who should return to have it checked in 24 hours).

The limb should be placed comfortably on a soft waterproof pillow ensuring that natural curves are supported. It should be exposed to the air for drying. It is not considered advisable to use artificial heat to hasten the drying process. Patient should be kept warm. 12 to 24 hours should be allowed for hardening of the plaster and even longer for large plasters. The limb should be kept elevated and weight bearing is not allowed for at least 24 hours. Joints outside the plaster should be exercised.

Note and report any of the following

Obvious tightness of plaster accompanied by swelling of digits, discolouration, e.g. exposed parts becoming blue or white, interference with sensation, e.g. complaint of 'pins and needles', fingers or toes feeling very cold to the touch, plaster becoming soft or cracked, staining through plaster.

COMPLAINT OF PAIN MUST NEVER BE IGNORED.

Special care should be taken

Avoid crumbs of plaster getting inside cast. Instruct patient not to use objects like knitting needles to relieve pressure, and not to push cotton wool in at the edges. Watch that children do not push coins or other objects inside. Ensure that patient can use bed pan or toilet without soiling the plaster, when hip spica or plaster jacket has been applied.

Traction

The use of traction plays a large part in the treatment of fractures and other orthopaedic conditions. This is a means by which a pulling force can be applied to a limb, the head and neck, or the pelvis, in its long axis.

Main purposes

To restore alignment of a fracture or dislocation.

To overcome spasm of muscle and relieve pain in diseases of joints or following injury.

To immobilise a limb or other part of the body such as the head and neck.

To help prevent deformity.

These can be achieved in the following ways:

1. Skeletal traction

The pull is applied directly to the skeleton by passing a metal pin or wire transversely through a bone, e.g. a Steinmann's pin passed through the upper end of the tibia in the treatment of a fractured shaft of femur. This is normally carried out in theatre under a general anaesthetic although it may be done in a treatment room in an emergency and using a local anaesthetic.

2. Skin traction

The pull is exerted through the skin by applying specially prepared orthopaedic adhesive material and attaching cords and weights. This permits a milder traction than skeletal and is used for shorter periods of time.

This may be applied by an experienced nurse.

The traction applied may be:

Fixed, e.g. using a Thomas' splint without pulleys or weights.

Balanced, e.g. using a Thomas' splint and pulleys and weights or raising the foot of the bed to provide counter traction.

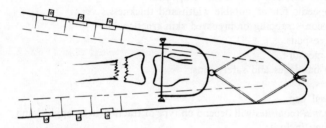

Figure 55.1
Fixed skeletal traction

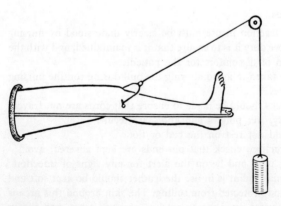

Figure 55.2
Balanced skeletal traction

Application of skin traction

Trolley with the following:

Requisites for shaving the skin.

Dressing pack with swabs, gallipot, dressing forceps and drape.

Bottle of tincture of benzoin compound.

Orthopaedic felt of suitable width and thickness.

Extension strapping or prepared skin traction kit.

Gamgee pads.

Tape measure.

Crepe bandages and safety pins.

Scissors.

Disposal bag.

Additional requisites will depend on type of traction to be applied and may include:

Thomas' splint and canvas slings or double tubigrip.

Spreader and extension cord.

Pulleys and weights.

Balkan beam.

Bed blocks or bed elevator.

Fracture boards are placed under the mattress and a bed cradle made available for use.

Clinical notes

Principles of traction in use must be clearly understood by nursing staff whose duty it is to ensure that it is maintained, and with the minimum of discomfort for the patient.

Care must be taken to avoid altering the pull during routine nursing procedures.

Frequent checks should be made to ensure that cords are not frayed, run freely over pulleys and knots are secure.

Weights should not rest on the bed or floor.

In skeletal traction, check that pin ends are kept covered, avoid touching pins, and be on the alert for any signs of infection.

When a Thomas' splint is in use the leather should be kept soft and pliable and protected from soiling. The skin around this area is given frequent attention to prevent pressure sores, and the patient instructed how to move the skin under the ring regularly.

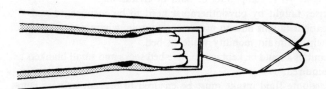

Figure 56.1
Fixed skin traction

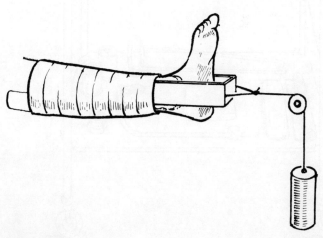

Figure 56.2
Balanced skin traction

Observation and treatment of all other areas which are at risk and where pressure sores may develop, including underneath the adhesive in skin traction.

Be on the alert for any impairment of circulation and report swelling, blueness, pallor or coldness of limbs.

Nerve pressure may result in complaint of 'pins and needles'.

Investigate ALL complaints of pain or irritation.

Exercises taught by physiotherapist need to be encouraged and patient taught how to use extension pole, where appropriate, to help maintain mobility while in bed.

Extremities should be kept warm. Use bed socks and small blankets as required.

An adequate fluid intake must be ensured to prevent urinary complications.

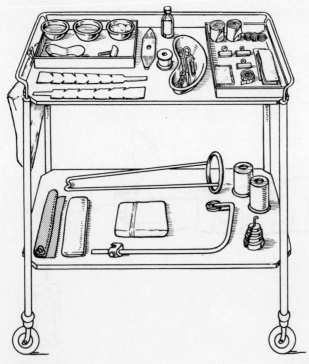

Figure 56.3
Trolley for application of skin traction

Help and support in the use of bed pans and attention to toilet needs is most important.

The use of aperients and suppositories may be necessary to ensure satisfactory bowel evacuation.

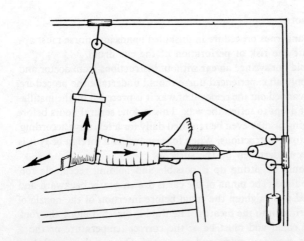

Figure 57
Hamilton-Russell type of traction (arrows indicate direction of pull)

Syringing an ear

This treatment may be prescribed for the removal of wax or an accumulation of moist keratin from the external auditory meatus. It may also be necessary for removal of certain types of foreign bodies.

Requirements

Tray or trolley with the following:

Receptacle with aural syringe (metal type or Higginson's bulb syringe with an aural tip attached).

Jug with the prescribed lotion at temperature 37.2°C. Lotion used may be a solution of saline or sodium bicarbonate.

Lotion thermometer.

Receptacle for returned lotion, e.g. kidney dish or ear trough.

Ear dressing pack containing cotton wool and applicators.

Auriscope or head mirror.

Aural speculum and forceps.

Anglepoise lamp.

Disposal bag.

Shoulder cape and disposable towel.

Clinical notes

This is a dangerous procedure in unskilled hands and nurse must appreciate the risk of perforation of the ear drum.

Nurse should not syringe an ear without instructions from doctor and then only an experienced nurse should undertake the procedure.

When it is carried out for removal of wax it is preceded by the instillation of drops to soften the wax. This is done several hours before syringing or may even be repeated daily for a few days according to doctor's instructions. When for removal of a foreign body it is usually undertaken by the surgeon.

Patient should be sitting up if possible and holding receptacle for return fluid. The pinna of the ear is drawn gently backward and upward to straighten the canal before insertion of the nozzle of the syringe into the meatus. The fluid is directed along the roof of the canal and must be at the correct temperature or the patient may feel giddy and nauseated. On completion of the irrigation the external canal must be thoroughly dried.

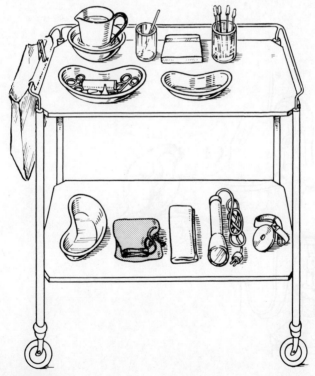

Figure 58
Trolley for syringing the ear

153

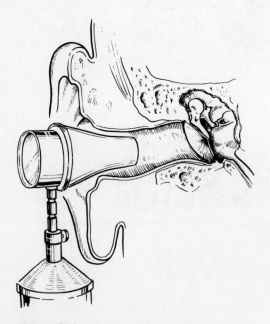

Figure 59.1
Examination of the ear using an auriscope

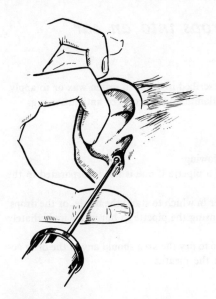

Figure 59.2
Retraction of the pinna (backwards and upwards)

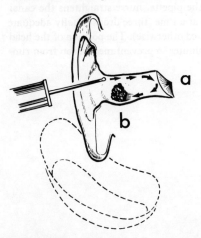

Figure 59.3
Direction of flow of solution when syringing the ear   a. tympanic membrane (ear drum)   b. wax in ear

Insertion of drops into an ear

This treatment may be prescribed in order to soften wax or to apply medication such as anti-inflammatory steroids or antibiotics, e.g. neomycin.

Requirements

A small tray with the following:

The prescribed drops, and a pipette if one is not incorporated in the stopper of the bottle.

A small bowl of warm water in which to stand the bottle, or the drops may be warmed by rinsing the pipette in hot water immediately before use.

A cotton wool mop or tissue to dry the area should any of the drug accidentally fall outside the meatus.

Clinical notes

The patient lies on his side with the ear to be treated uppermost or is seated with the head tilted to the unaffected side.

Having drawn the drug into the pipette, nurse straightens the canal and inserts the drops one at a time (three drops usually adequate unless specifically instructed otherwise). The position of the head is maintained for a few minutes to prevent medication from running out of the ear.

Insertion of a wick into an ear

This is an alternative method of applying medication to the ear by using a length of ribbon gauze which may be impregnated with an ointment or soaked in lotion in a small gallipot.

Requirements

A small tray with the following:
Ribbon gauze.
Prescribed medication and small bowl.
Aural dressing forceps.
Head mirror.

Clinical notes

Position patient as before and ensure a good light.
Gently insert the prepared gauze into the meatus using aural dressing forceps.
Care must be taken to ensure that it is folded into the meatus loosely and not packed tightly.
It should reach the end of the canal close to the tympanic membrane (7.5 cm is usually adequate).

Notes

Instillation of nasal drops

The commonest preparations used are vaso-constrictors such as ephedrine or tuamine sulphate.

Requirements

A small tray with:

The prescribed drops (slightly warmed by standing the bottle in a small bowl of warm water).

A disposable pipette.

Tissues and a sputum carton.

Disposable drape.

Clinical notes

If necessary the nostrils are cleaned before commencing.

It may suffice for the patient to blow the nose.

Patient is placed in the supine position with a pillow under the shoulders only or the head over the edge of the bed or couch.

The drops are drawn up into the pipette and instilled a drop at a time into one nostril and then the other. Approximately 3 or 4 drops for each nostril.

Patient is asked to breathe through the mouth during the procedure.

Tissues are used to wipe away any excess as position is changed and a sputum carton should be available to allow patient to spit out any that may have run down into the oro-pharynx.

Notes

Tracheostomy

A tracheostomy is a temporary or permanent opening made into the trachea in order to establish satisfactory ventilation and permit of tracheo-bronchial suction.

Indications for the procedure

When airway obstruction is likely to occur or has already occurred, including:

1. Laryngeal obstruction which may be due to oedema of the glottis, an impacted foreign body or acute laryngo-tracheo-bronchitis, especially in children.
2. As a preliminary to operations, e.g. laryngectomy.
3. Paralysis of the vocal cords, e.g. after partial thyroidectomy.
4. Tumours of the larynx.
5. Management of the unconscious patient, e.g. following head injuries.
6. Paralysis in poliomyelitis.

The insertion of the tracheostomy tube may be a *planned operation* under general anaesthesia *or a life-saving emergency* measure with or without the use of a local anaesthetic.

After-care of a tracheostomy

A trolley which is cleaned and disinfected as for all sterile procedures is kept at the bedside with requisites for attention to dressings, changing of tracheostomy tube, and facilitation of suction.

An exact replica of the tracheostomy tube used (with tapes). See Figure 60.2.

Supply of sterile gloves.

Sterile tracheostomy dressing pack containing cotton wool mops, gauze swabs, gallipot, 3 pairs non-toothed dissecting forceps and 2 pieces of tape.

Sterile sodium bicarbonate solution and foil bowl.

Packet with sterile disposable catheters for suction.

1 pair tracheal dilators.

1 pair pointed scissors.

Syringe and adaptor when a cuffed tracheostomy tube is used.

A disposal bag for soiled dressings.

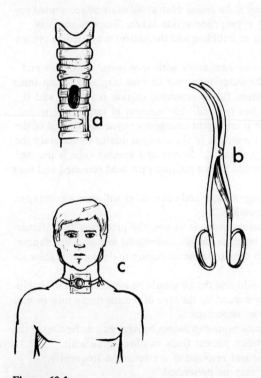

Figure 60.1
a. Tracheostomy site   b. tracheal dilators   c. tube in position and secured with tapes tied round neck

A receptacle for soiled non-disposable equipment.
An antiseptic lotion, e.g. solution of Hibitane (aqueous).
Oxygen and special tracheostomy mask when necessary.
Suction apparatus or 'piped' suction available.

Clinical notes

Patient is nursed semi-recumbent or in the sitting position unless this
is contra-indicated by general condition.

The tube must remain patent and nurse should know how to carry out
regular cleansing and application of suction when necessary.

All aseptic precautions must be taken to prevent tracheostomy infection.

Signs that the airway is becoming obstructed must be recognised immediately and appropriate action taken. Respirations may
become rattling or bubbling and the patient may become cyanosed.

The tube may become obstructed with secretions, blood clot and
crusting, or the outer tube may become displaced. If an inner
tube is in position this is removed, suction is applied and if
obstruction is not relieved, displacement of outer tube is
suspected. This is an urgent emergency requiring removal of the
outer tube and insertion of the tracheal dilator to maintain the
opening until medical aid arrives and another tube is inserted.
(The patient should be in a position with head retracted and neck
extended.)

The routine changing of inner and outer tubes will vary according to
surgeon's instructions.

If a cuffed tracheostomy tube is in use, the procedure for inflation
and deflation must be clearly understood and also the dangers
associated with over inflation or failure to deflate at regular intervals.

Some means of humidifying the air should be available and the equipment used may depend on the type of tracheostomy tube *in situ*.

Oral hygiene is most important.

Nutritional needs may require to be met by naso-gastric feeding in the
initial stages when patient finds swallowing difficult.

Temperature, pulse and respiration are recorded frequently.

Antibiotic therapy may be prescribed.

Regular turning and chest physiotherapy are important.

When patient is conscious a pencil and paper should be provided for
communication and a bell or other means of summoning nurse
should be available.

Information, advice and support for relatives as well as patient is
vitally important.

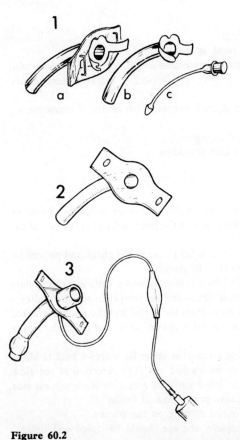

Figure 60.2
Types of tracheostomy tubes 1. Jackson's metal tube a. outer tube b. inner tube c. introducer 2. Plastic tube 3. Plastic (cuffed) tube

Irrigation of eye

This treatment may be ordered:

For removal of chemicals which have been splashed on the eye.
As part of routine preparation for operation.
For removal of a foreign body which is not embedded.

Requirements

Tray with the following:
A sterile undine in a bowl or stand.
A jug containing 300 ml of prescribed lotion, e.g. sterile saline solution temperature 37.7°C, and cooled to suitable temperature before use.
Fisher's dish or kidney shaped receptacle for return of irrigation lotion.
Eye pack with sterile dressings.
Waterproof cape to protect shoulders.
Disposal bag.

Clinical notes

Patient should be seated comfortably in a chair with a head rest, or lying in a supine position with the head inclined to the side of the eye being treated.

The dish for return of lotion is held close to the cheek and patient instructed how to hold it in position.

Patient is warned when lotion is coming and a little is directed onto the cheek first so that he can feel the temperature. The undine is held about 2.5 cm away from the eyelid and the patient is asked to look up as the lower lid is drawn down and the lower fornix irrigated.

The patient next looks down and the upper lid is drawn back to allow the upper fornix to be washed out. The direction of the flow should be from the inner canthus across to the temporal side, maintaining a steady, gentle flow of lotion.

Lotion must not be poured directly on the cornea.

When irrigation is complete, the eye should be closed and dried carefully with sterile cotton wool mops.

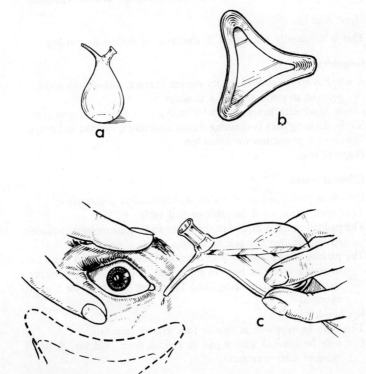

Figure 61
Irrigation of the eye
a. undine   b. Fisher's irrigation tray   c. lotion allowed to flow on cheek
before being directed into lower fornix

Application of heat to the eye

This may be prescribed to:
Relieve pain, increase the blood supply or hasten the absorption of drugs.

Dry heat

This may be applied using a small electric pad, the Maddox heater. It may be used for one hour in four and the amount of heat regulated.

Moist heat

This is frequently prescribed in the form of *hot spoon bathing*.

Requirements

A wooden spoon padded on its convex surface with cotton wool secured in position with a bandage.
Lotion bowl with hot water and standing in a deep treatment tray.
Sterile dressing pack containing cotton wool mops, eye pad and drape.
Waterproof protection for shoulders.
Disposal bag.

Clinical notes

Patient is positioned comfortably with shoulders protected.
Tray with lotion bowl on table or bed table.
The padded spoon is dipped in the water and excess moisture squeezed out against the side of bowl.
The patient leans forward, head over bowl, eye closed, and holds the steaming spoon as near to the eyelid as possible but does not touch eye or surrounding skin. Treatment continued for 5 to 10 minutes.
Eyelids dried.
This may be repeated at two to four hourly intervals.
Eye may be covered with a pad to protect from cold for 20 to 30 minutes after treatment.

Eye bathing

Indications for treatment

The need to remove exudate or crusts prior to further treatment.
Care of the eyes in unconscious patient where the corneal reflex is
lost.
Any condition causing excessive drying of eyes.

Requirements

Tray with the following:
Jug with sterile solution, e.g. sodium bicarbonate or saline,
temperature 37.7°C.
Sterile eye pack containing cotton wool mops, gallipot and drape.
Disposal bag.
Add a bottle of olive oil and an additional gallipot when required, for
removal of ointment which has been previously applied to the
lids.

Clinical notes

Nurse should stand behind the patient or at the side of the eye being
treated.
The patient is asked to look up while the lower lid is drawn down and
swabbed gently, then he looks down while the upper lid is everted
and swabbed in the same way.
Each swab is used ONCE only.
Swabbing is from within outwards.
Care must be taken to ensure that neither swabs nor fingers touch the
cornea.

Notes

Instillation of eye drops

This may be necessary

As a prophylactic measure or in the treatment of infection, when an antibiotic may be prescribed.

To dilate the pupil (mydriatic drops), e.g. prior to ophthalmoscopic examination of the fundus.

To contract the pupil (miotic drops), e.g. to reduce tension in treatment of glaucoma.

To anaesthetise the eye before surgery or certain treatments such as removal of solid caustic material.

Requirements

Patient's prescription card.

Bottle with eye drops and a sterile disposable dropper or a sterile single dose unit may be available.

Cotton wool mop.

Clinical notes

Special care must be taken to check the written prescription against the drops to be used, the patient's name, and the eye to be treated, i.e. right or left.

Checking and administration should be witnessed by a second person when necessary.

If a bottle with a pipette is used measures must be taken to prevent it touching any part of the eye and thus becoming contaminated.

Nurse should stand behind the patient or at the side of the eye being treated, support the head well back with the chin up.

Patient is asked to look up and the lower lid is gently retracted just before the drop is instilled on to the lower fornix, the dropper being held 2.5 cm away from the eye.

Always warn patient before drop is instilled.

Eyelids closed gently and dried if necessary.

It is important to prevent any drops falling on the skin or into the opposite eye.

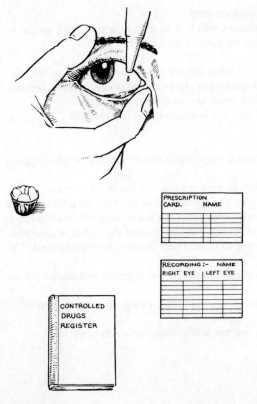

Figure 62
Instillation of eye drops. Enter in 'controlled drugs' register when necessary

Application of ointment to the eye

Indications for this treatment

Prevention of spread of infection in hordeolum (stye).
Conjunctivitis.
Blepharitis.
Prevention of symblepharon (adhesion of the lid to the globe).

Requirements

The patient's prescription card.
The prescribed ointment which is usually in a tube with specially
   designed nozzle for ease of application.
Cotton wool.
A sterile glass eye rod when the method of application is to be 'rod-
   ding'. The rod must always be examined to ensure that it is quite
   smooth and free from any roughness or chips.
(Applicaps, single dose eye ointments may be available).

Clinical notes

The eye is first bathed as required, to remove exudate or crusting, and
   gently dried.
The patient is asked to look up and the lower lid is pulled down.
A little ointment may be squeezed from the tube directly into the
   lower fornix, taking care that the nozzle does not touch the eye.
Alternatively, the ointment is squeezed onto the end of a glass rod,
   which is then placed in the lower fornix (horizontally inside the
   lower lid).
The patient closes the eyes and the rod is gently withdrawn via the
   outer canthus.
The eyelids may be gently massaged, except in a post-operative
   patient.
Check that lashes are not stuck down with ointment.

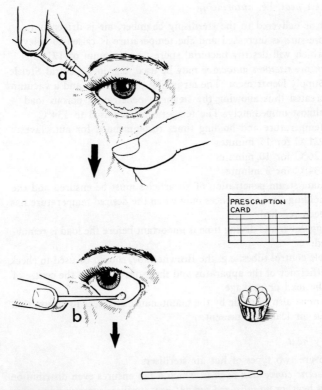

PRESCRIPTION
CARD

Figure 63
Application of ointment to the eye   a. directly from a tube   b. using a glass
rod

Sterilisation

This may be defined as the removal or destruction of all living microbes, i.e. bacteria, viruses, protozoa and fungi (and includes bacterial spores).

There are several methods in common use.

Heat

1. *Moist heat*, i.e. *autoclaving*

Steam is delivered to the sterilising chamber, air is driven out, pressure is increased and the temperature is raised to a level which will destroy bacterial spores, a minimum of 121°C.

A high pre-vacuum autoclave may be used, e.g. in a Central Sterile Supply Department. The air is first pumped out and a vacuum created thus allowing the steam to penetrate a porous load almost immediately. The temperature is raised to 134°C.

The temperature and holding times recommended for autoclaves:

121°C for 15 minutes
126°C for 10 minutes
134°C for 3 minutes

Adequate steam penetration of all articles must be ensured and the holding time commences only when the desired temperature has been reached.

Cooling down and drying time is important before the load is removed.

Reliable control tubes, e.g. the Browne tube, should be used to check efficiency of the apparatus and these are placed in the centre of the load or package.

Tests must also be made by the maintenance engineer to ensure that no air leaks are present.

2. *Dry heat*

There are two types of hot air sterilisers.

An electric convection oven in which a fan ensures even distribution of heat, or an *infra-red radiant heat* steriliser surrounding a conveyer belt and operating at a much higher temperature for a shorter exposure time.

The high temperature reached makes these methods of sterilisation unsuitable for many materials, e.g. dressings, cloth, paper, rubber, plastic, etc.

Their use is therefore more limited than the autoclave.

The temperature and holding times recommended for hot air ovens.

160°C for 45 minutes

170°C for 18 minutes

180°C for 7 minutes 30 seconds

190°C for 1 minute 30 seconds

All articles to be sterilised by heat should be suitable for the method which is used and care must be taken to ensure that the process is carried out properly.

In most hospitals sterilisation is centralised in special departments and is the responsibility of a team of skilled technicians.

Other sterilisation techniques

Gamma-radiation. Equipment necessary for this method of sterilisation remains extremely costly and is unsuitable for use in hospitals. An increasing number of commercially supplied disposable items are sterilised by the use of gamma rays from a radioactive source. Syringes, needles, catheters, tubing and many heat-sensitive materials are treated in this way.

Low temperature steam and formaldehyde. This method of sterilising heat-sensitive materials employs low temperature steam at subatmospheric pressure together with formaldehyde vapour.

A modification in design and operation of a high pre-vacuum autoclave allows for exposure of the materials to a mixture of steam and formaldehyde at 80°C. The recommended holding time is two hours.

Problems of toxicity are minimal.

Ethylene oxide. Sterilisation by exposure to ethylene oxide gas requires expensive apparatus. The whole operation must be under the control of specially qualified staff. The gas mixture used, the temperature reached and the time of the sterilising cycle varies with the type of machine in use.

Problems may arise with the possibility of toxic residue in processed items and control of humidity. The effectiveness of the process is monitored by a bacteriologist. It is used for a number of heat-sensitive materials.

Disinfection

This may be defined as the removal or destruction of harmful
microbes, not usually or necessarily including bacterial spores.
The differentiation between 'sterilisation' and 'disinfection' should be
understood by all nurses.
In practice there are situations which require the use of a sterilisation
process e.g., dressings, syringes, needles and all instruments used
in surgical work must be sterile. There are other situations where
the use of a reliable disinfection process will have the desired
effect, i.e. of rendering articles safe to handle or use and also of
satisfactorily disinfecting the skin or mucous membranes.

Heat: pasteurization

This method is widely used in hospital for disinfection of bedpans,
linen, crockery, anaesthetic equipment, resuscitation apparatus
and instruments, e.g. cystoscopes.
The equipment used may be:
1. *A hot water pasteurizer* which is filled with water and loaded with
the equipment to be disinfected. The most satisfactory type has a
pre-set process timer, and an automatic pilot switch which indicates when the equipment may be removed. The temperature
and the holding time will vary, e.g.
Instruments 65 to 75°C for 10 minutes
Bedpan washers 80°C for 1 to 2 minutes
Articles for pasteurization should always be cleaned thoroughly
before this process is commenced.
Some items of equipment are dealt with in apparatus which is specially designed to combine washing with pasteurization.
In emergencies an ordinary boiler or suitable container may be used
in which equipment can be boiled (100°C for 5 minutes) but this
is not considered a satisfactory procedure in hospital.
2. *A steam pasteurizer*. This is a specially designed unit which
provides for exposure to steam at 70 to 80°C and is considered a
most suitable method of disinfection.
Temperature and holding times are adjusted as required, 70°C for 15
minutes or 80°C for 5 minutes.

A modified high pre-vacuum autoclave operating at sub-atmospheric pressure will provide steam at 80°C and an exposure time of 5 minutes will be sufficient to disinfect. (This is the type of equipment used in conjunction with formaldehyde vapour for sterilisation of some heat-sensitive materials.)

Chemicals

There is an extremely wide range of chemical disinfectants available and those used in hospital should be chosen on the basis of available scientific evidence.

The following should be clearly understood when deciding which disinfectant to recommend in any particular circumstances:

Its antimicrobial properties.

The concentration in which it has proved effective.

The minimum contact period required for satisfactory disinfection.

A number of variables must be considered, e.g. the type of contamination, the material to be disinfected and the accessibility of the bacteria. It must also be borne in mind that the presence of organic material will reduce effectiveness and necessitate a longer contact period than for a clean surface.

Any risks involved such as injury to skin or other tissues.

Possible adverse effects on equipment which may result from too high concentration or unnecessarily prolonged exposure.

Conditions which inactivate, e.g. soap will inactivate cetrimide/chlorhexidine which is frequently added to bath water as a precaution against staphylococcal infection.

The value of routine 'in-use' testing of disinfectants cannot be over-emphasised. This requires the co-operation of all concerned in preparation, use and monitoring of the effectiveness of the disinfectants which are being used.

It has been recommended that the use of chemical disinfectants be kept to a minimum but the following are in common use in hospitals:

Isopropyl alcohol

Chlorhexidine (Hibitane) – alcoholic or aqueous

Clearsol

Savlon

Cetavlon

Betadine

Dettol – and many others.

Each hospital or group of hospitals may have its own policy regarding disinfectants which may be supplied for use. The recommended concentrations will be outlined in the policy and the manufacturers also provide a guide for users of their products.

Some general rules regarding sterile equipment

Care must be taken with storage and handling of all sterile packs.
They should be kept in a clean, dry storage area or cupboard.
Special dispensing units which facilitate the use of equipment in proper rotation may be provided.
If the outer wrapping of a pre-sterilised pack is damaged in any way the contents will not be sterile.
Pre-sterilised disposables must be discarded after use and no attempt should be made to re-sterilise.
Special care should be exercised with disposal of syringes and needles which are of the disposable type.
If equipment is not disposable and is to be re-sterilized for further use it should be discarded immediately into the appropriate container which may be the pack from which it was removed or a receptacle containing a solution of a chemical disinfectant.

Index